Neuropsychosocial Intervention

The Practical Treatment of Severe Behavioral Dyscontrol after Acquired Brain Injury

Neuropsychosocial Intervention

The Practical Treatment of Severe Behavioral Dyscontrol after Acquired Brain Injury

ROBERT L. KAROL

CRC PRESS

Boca Raton London New York Washington, D.C.

Library of Congress Cataloging-in-Publication Data

Karol, Robert L.
Neuropsychosocial intervention : the practical treatment of severe behavioral dyscontrol after acquired brain injury / Robert L. Karol.
p. cm.
Includes bibliographical references and index.
ISBN 0-8493-1244-2 (alk. paper)
1. Brain damage—Patients—Rehabilitation. 2. Combined modality therapy. 3. Psychology, Pathological. I. Title.

RC387.5.K376 2003
616.8′043—dc21 2003043492

Direct all inquiries to CRC Press LLC, 2000 N.W. Corporate Blvd., Boca Raton, Florida 33431.

International Standard Book Number 0-8493-1244-2
Library of Congress Card Number 2003043492
Printed in the United States of America 1 2 3 4 5 6 7 8 9 0
Printed on acid-free paper

Dedication

for

Gwendolyn Barnes-Karol, with love forever and ever.

No manner of written communication can convey the debt I owe her or the admiration I hold for her. She is brilliant and selfless. Yet, she asks for no recognition. Her greatest satisfaction comes from helping others. She is naturally empathic. She holds my soul together.

Preface

Motor vehicle accidents. Falls down stairs. Sports collisions. Strokes. Falls off ladders. Drug overdoses. Heart attacks. Muggings. Near drownings. In a brief moment, sometimes a split second, a person's concerns about tomorrow change from the groceries, the rent, a date, mowing the lawn, a promotion, or paying the bills to survival. And then the groceries, the rent ... become important again. Except this time, one has cognitive problems and cannot remember important concerns or one has emotional difficulties and is depressed and irritable.

Beyond these symptoms of cognitive deficits and emotional challenges lies behavioral dyscontrol. Behavioral dyscontrol cannot be ignored, because it interferes with all other treatment and any possibility of success in life after brain injury. Yet behavioral dyscontrol is the problem therapists, families, and persons with brain injury find the most difficult to address. Most therapists are poorly prepared to treat behavioral dyscontrol, particularly when it is severe in nature. Hence, persons with brain injury who exhibit severe behavioral problems may be locked in jail or state hospitals.

This book describes an intervention methodology to address behavioral dyscontrol, even when the behavior is severe. The therapy is called neuropsychosocial treatment. Neuropsychosocial treatment changes the world to fit the needs of persons with brain injury. It is an environmental intervention that focuses on the behavior of the people whom persons with brain injury encounter and the physical environment that they inhabit. Therapists create this environment after they formulate an understanding of the phenomenology of behavioral dyscontrol for each person with brain injury based upon an examination of neurological, cognitive, adjustment, and environmental variables.

The treatment model this book describes differs from traditional interventions in two ways. First, construction of a new environment *is* the treatment. In traditional treatment, environmental manipulation is used for insight acquisition, skill building, or contingency management. Second, neuropsychosocial intervention works even when the above therapies fail.

This book describes procedures that are based on over 20 years of clinical work with persons with brain injury, 10 of those years specializing in the treatment of behavioral dyscontrol. During that time, the treatment methodology that this book details has been used to successfully address very severe behavioral dyscontrol by persons with brain injury. Persons with brain injury are living in the community today, rather than in jail or a state hospital, because of neuropsychosocial intervention. This book offers therapists a methodology for treatment that works, even with seemingly intractable cases. Of course, therapists may also find the information here helpful to treat less severe behavioral dyscontrol, either alone or in conjunction with traditional therapies.

This book provides an integrated approach for the treatment of behavioral dyscontrol. In contrast, behavioral management techniques are usually presented as a list of strategies as if they were items on a menu. The author of this book believes that such a cookbook approach fails to give therapists guidance in how to organize treatment. For this reason, this book rebalances case conceptualization and techniques. The usual presentation of behavioral interventions focuses on interventions that are too simplistic for true cases of severe behavioral dyscontrol. The author has seen an overwhelming number of cases where therapists have applied various simplistic behavioral strategies, often documented in detailed behavioral management plans numerous pages in length, that do not work. These plans either lack an overall case conceptualization or consist of behavioral tactics that are inadequate. This book, in contrast, presents an integrated approach that includes treatment philosophy and concrete application.

In addition, this book includes discussion of professional issues for therapists who work with persons with brain injury who exhibit behavioral dyscontrol. The application of any behavioral treatment requires very skillful therapists. These therapists face continual professional and emotional hurdles, as treating severe behavioral dyscontrol is difficult work. However, too often, behavioral interventions are presented as if they were a matter of simply implementing textbook tactics. Then, treatment fails when therapists ignore real-world case issues such as treatment setbacks, disruptive families, therapists being hit, team discord, financial concerns, confusion about professional roles, etc. This book interweaves discussion of such issues into the material on clinical work.

Chapter 1 presents the neuropsychosocial approach and outlines its parameters. It contrasts this approach with traditional treatment procedures, noting the problems that therapists have when applying traditional interventions for persons with brain injury. It also discusses the social penalty of inadequate treatment of behavioral dyscontrol.

Chapter 2 reviews cognitive variables that therapists must consider in order to understand behavioral dyscontrol. Too often, therapists devise behavioral plans without careful consideration of cognitive data. Therefore, the emphasis in this chapter is a clinical one: how to link knowledge about cognitive deficits to observed behavioral dyscontrol.

Chapter 3 discusses adjustment factors that have an impact on behavioral dyscontrol. The chapter relates issues of adjustment directly to behavioral dyscontrol. The intent is for therapists to accurately consider adjustment variables that influence the expression of behavioral dyscontrol.

In Chapter 4, therapists will learn the importance of integrating all information at their disposal into a conceptualization of behavioral dyscontrol for each person with brain injury. The chapter discusses the types of team functioning that facilitate the ability of therapists to accurately conceptualize raw observations. Finally, the chapter presents common phenomenological variables that therapists are likely to encounter as they integrate cognitive and emotional data.

Dr. Laura McDaniels provides concrete core behavior plans in Chapter 5. These plans give therapists a place to start for 18 typical problem behaviors. They are intended as initial departure points from which therapists can construct individualized neuropsychosocial environments. In this chapter, Dr. McDaniels also discusses some common modifications of the core plans.

Dr. Robert Sevenich discusses the integration of medication management and neuropsychosocial treatment in Chapter 6. This chapter provides valuable information on an integrated approach for therapists and physicians alike. This chapter will help nonphysician therapists design behavioral treatment with consideration of both the benefit of pharmacological intervention on behavioral dyscontrol and the impact of medications on the application of behavioral treatment. Similarly, this chapter will assist physicians in adequately adjusting medication in light of behavioral plan implementation. Furthermore, Dr. Sevenich reviews specific classes of medications from a clinical perspective as they relate to behavioral management after brain injury.

Chapter 7 tackles the challenge of community placement. First, it addresses the crucial concept of feeling dependent that persons with brain injury must confront. Then, it reviews why there is an inadequate supply of residential options. Next, this chapter reviews how placement sites need to function to handle behavioral concerns and to implement a neuropsychosocial environment. Chapter 7 ends with a discussion of variables that therapists need to consider when preparing to handle episodes of aggression. Therapists need to be ready if their behavioral management plan does not work in every instance. This chapter guides therapists in preparing for unexpected events.

Finally, Chapter 8 presents clinical scenarios that highlight the application of the neuropsychosocial approach. These vignettes bring to life how therapists can assess and conceptualize behavioral dyscontrol and then devise treatment. The vignettes are intended to let therapists see how the process of neuropsychosocial treatment takes shape.

This book was written with the intent of filling a gap in the treatment of behavioral dyscontrol after brain injury. The author's hope is that therapists who apply neuropsychosocial treatment will expand their current armamentarium for addressing behavioral dyscontrol. They will have a coherent way to conceptualize treatment. They will be prepared to integrate cognitive and adjustment variables into a comprehensive model of a phenomenology of behavioral dyscontrol for each case. Therapists will be able to develop and apply concrete behavior plans while considering the advantages of coordinated medication management. Such an approach will enable therapists to apply their expertise in community settings. Finally, they will be better prepared if everything does not work perfectly.

When this book was conceived, it was designed to appeal to a wide range of therapists and others concerned about the need of persons with brain injury to have good behavioral performance. The book's intent is to help psychologists, neuropsychologists, nurses, occupational therapists, physical therapists, speech and language pathologists, behavioral analysts, chaplains, recreational therapists, and other therapists design better treatment. Its goal is also to give physicians information to better integrate their knowledge with behavioral intervention. For social workers, case managers, and third-party representatives, this book should provide insight into what is possible in behavioral management with their assistance as well as what is not feasible. Finally, for family members and persons with brain injury, this book should give hope, tempered by realism. With your help, there is a treatment methodology that works.

Robert L. Karol
Bethesda Rehabilitation Hospital

Acknowledgments

Books always represent the combined effort of numerous people, a point with which I became reacquainted on almost a daily basis as I wrote this book. Sadly, acknowledgements inadequately capture the debt I owe so many people. So, to all the following people, I am sorry that the words here cannot do justice to the feelings I have for all of you who contributed to the creation of this book. Your support was crucial to my being able to complete this book and enjoy the experience.

Foremost in my mind are all the persons with brain injury who have taught me about brain injury. I am better able to help other persons with brain injury because of the wisdom I have gained over the years from persons with brain injury about what works and what does not work. In essence, therapists are a conduit of accumulated experience from many past clients to the next person needing help. With this in mind, I hope that this book will further pass on that accumulated knowledge.

It is impossible for me to contemplate persons with brain injury without recognizing the Brain Injury Association of Minnesota. Over the years, the volunteers, staff, and members of the Board of Directors have contributed greatly to my perspectives on persons with brain injury. I wish to acknowledge the impact on me of Fran Conklin, Chris Duff, Baba Finch, Tom Gode, Ellie Hands, Robin Landy, Craig Martinson, Katie O'Brien, Dr. Bill O'Dowd, Chuck Ramsbacher, Ardis Sandstrom, and Dr. Carole Wedel Sellars.

I have also had the advantage of working with excellent people at the Minnesota Department of Human Services; in particular, Sharyl Helgeson and Michelle Long. The ideas in this book are mine, not theirs, but our discussions, both agreements and disagreements, have been very important to me. Also, I want to recognize Mark Kinde at the Minnesota Department of Health for his efforts in data collection on behalf of persons with brain injury.

Kerry Burak and Lori Huffman have my gratitude for providing background information and thoughts about community placements. They are very experienced and knowledgeable. Of course, I take full responsibility for my interpretation of the information they provided.

I have benefited greatly from my professional association with organizations and people who have contributed to my knowledge of the challenges that persons with brain injury face. These include Marty Cushing, Greg Jones, Duane Reynolds, Sue Rivard, Beth Skwira, TBI Metro Services, and Vinland Center. In addition, Cleone Brazil gave me amazing professional support early in my career and helped shape my thoughts about brain injury. Garry Woessner also has my respect for his insights into brain injury care. Our too infrequent conversations are always a source of enlightenment for me.

Recognition is also due my colleagues at Karol Neuropsychological Services & Consulting: Dr. Nancy Carlson, Dr. Bridget Hegeman, and Dr. Thomas Kern. Their reflections are invaluable and their hard work energizes me.

This book would have been impossible without the assistance of everyone at Bethesda Rehabilitation Hospital. At Bethesda, all the therapists, in the broadest sense of the word as used in this book, are the champions behind this book. It is impossible to list everyone, as it would take a few hundred pages. However, thanks are due everyone who works in Brain Injury Services on our hospital units and on our Green and Purple Teams.

Still, I would like to specifically acknowledge certain people. To start, I am blessed by the support of a spectacular team of psychologists: Dr. Cheri Brunetti, Dr. Laurie Dunn, Dr. Maida Gunther, Dr. Kristi Hyink-Huttemier, Dr. Laura McDaniels, Dr. Linda Rickard, and Dr. Jane Siegal. They perform daily miracles supporting people confronting otherwise overwhelming illnesses and injuries. They do so with ongoing dedication and empathy. They are a wonderful team.

Similarly, I receive encouragement from every member of our medical staff. Every single physician is personally committed to our hospital at a level rarely seen. Dr. Robert Sevenich, our psychiatrist, and Dr. Kenneth Britton, our physiatrist, deserve special recognition for their work with persons with brain injury. They also routinely attend rounds *together*, an asset beyond belief for brain injury care. Therapists in many other settings rarely see such supradisciplinary medicine openly practiced live. Also, Dr. Charles Ormiston has my thanks for his early work in our program and for his ongoing support.

The treatment of severe behavioral dyscontrol after brain injury would be impossible without administrative encouragement. Our current and past administrators, Scott Batulis, Ross Huttunen, Dr. Frank Indihar, and Diana Johnson are committed to our programs for brain injury care. I could not offer the treatment that this book describes without their backing.

When episodes of behavioral dyscontrol occur in the community, referral sources tend to be desperate. All our admission coordinators deserve credit for balancing bed availability with the needs of referral sources, insurers, families, and persons with brain injury. I admire the work these coordinators all do. Of particular note, Sharon Malinowski is continually on the phone juggling competing demands with unbelievable tolerance. Admission to our programs and clinical excellence is only part of the story. Our case resource specialist, Micki Shaefer, and our social workers, Dorothy Connell, Char Elioff, and Sheryl Rorvig ensure that we use our time with persons with brain injury wisely and in a fashion that will lead to community placement. I appreciate their perspectives.

Lia Christiansen, De Granstrom, and Kim Harju deserve special mention for their help in my efforts to provide the community with education regarding brain injury. Mike Sandman and Bill Findorff have my praise for their dedication to the care of persons with brain injury. They routinely challenge my concepts and help make them better.

A number of people provided me with technical assistance. Linda Kojetin, Laura Moyer, Judy Taplin, and Lenida Sandahl struggled mightily to type my illegible handwritten drafts. Pat Radke helps make everything I need happen.

Amy Fehrer was a godsend locating reference material for this book, and in our clinical work she is invaluable in coordinating data collection on episodes of behavioral dyscontrol and medication administration to enhance our care of persons with brain injury. I also want to acknowledge Dorothy Cotton and Laurie Bane for their assistance with data collection and for keeping our clinical work organized.

I also owe heartfelt thanks to the people at CRC Press. They agreed to accept this book for publication when it was written only in my head, but not on paper. Then they helped me produce a book far beyond my abilities alone. I wish to recognize Carol Hollander, Barbara Ellen Norwitz, Tanya Li, Athalia Lujo, Patricia Roberson, Amy Rodriguez, Dawn Snyder, and Carolyn Spence. In addition, thanks are due Dr. Greg Hauge, Dr. Renee Hudson, and Dr. Greg Sitka. They offered encouragement when this book was being conceptualized.

So many brain injuries are preventable; people drive recklessly, take foolish risks in pursuit of excitement, use drugs, and assault each other. There are four people, however, who give me hope by their nature that people can be kinder to one other and can live more intelligently: Bradley, Daniel, Hilleary, and Meredith.

There is no work that I do that should omit appreciation of Patricia Florio, my second-grade teacher at Longfellow Elementary School in Teaneck, New Jersey. She saved me. In addition, my mother, Rhona, instilled in me an enduring concern for the well being of others that is reflected in the content of this book and in my clinical work.

And then there is Gwen. She encouraged me to pursue writing this book, and she took care of all my needs while I did so. She gave me emotional sustenance when I felt overwhelmed by grammar problems or when I panicked about deadlines. Moreover, in an effort beyond imagination, she read drafts of every chapter providing extraordinary assistance to me and my contributors. No one would know half as well what the author of this book was trying to say if it were not for her.

Robert L. Karol
St. Paul, Minnesota

About the Author

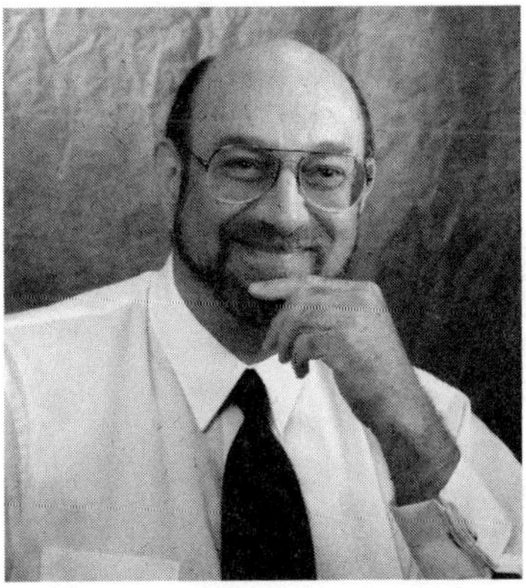

Robert L. Karol, Ph.D. is the program director of Brain Injury Services and director of Neuropsychology/Psychology at Bethesda Rehabilitation Hospital, in St. Paul, Minnesota. Brain Injury Services specializes in the treatment of behavioral dyscontrol after brain injury even for persons with brain injury who have failed other programs. He is the program chair for an annual conference: Managing Challenging Situations in Brain Injury Care. Dr. Karol heads a group private practice, Karol Neuropsychological Services & Consulting, in Minneapolis, Minnesota, specializing in neuropsychological evaluations and counseling for persons with brain injury, and he is a co-owner of Neuroscience Multispecialty Advisors, PLLC, a group including neurology, physiatry, psychiatry, gerontology, and neuropsychology that provides case consultation to lawyers and insurance companies.

Co-founder of the Brain Injury Association of Minnesota, Dr. Karol was a member of its board of directors for 14 years, and he is a past chairman of the board. He has served on the advisory committee for TBI Metro Services, which provides brain injury vocational services, and on the board of directors of Accessible Space, Inc., which provides brain injury residential programming. In addition, he has been on the Minnesota Department of Human Services Traumatic Brain Injury Program Advisory Committee for 10 years. Dr. Karol is a member of the Supreme Court of Minnesota's Board of Law Examiners' Special Test Accommodation Panel and is a consultant for Vinland Center's Brain Injury Chemical Dependency Program.

Dr. Karol earned his undergraduate degree at the University of Colorado at Boulder in psychology in 1974, and his doctorate from the University of Missouri at Columbia in clinical psychology in 1981. He is currently at work on research regarding the outcome of treatment for behavioral dyscontrol after acquired brain injury. He has conducted over 75 seminars, lectures, and workshops. In his free time, Dr. Karol is an avid chess player.

Contributors

Laura A. McDaniels, Psy.D.
Bethesda Rehabilitation Hospital
St. Paul, Minnesota

Robert Sevenich, M.D., J.D.
Brain Injury Services
Bethesda Rehabilitation Hospital
St. Paul, Minnesota

Contents

Terminology

Throughout this book, the author uses the term "persons with brain injury." The evolution of thought regarding appropriate terminology in this regard is interesting. It reflects an increasing awareness on the part of therapists of the importance of recognizing that persons with brain injury are people first. In fact, they may have many attributes that are more essential to knowing who they are as people than are their brain injuries, particularly in cases of milder brain injuries.

Therapists who have worked in the field of brain injury for some time can recall when the term "brain damaged" was the common term for a person following injury to the brain. Many therapists and persons with brain injury, however, felt that this term was demeaning. As a result, the term "head injured" emerged as a less offensive alternative. In fact, the Brain Injury Association of America began life as the National Head Injury Foundation. Yet, use of the term head injury gave rise to the public perception of such injuries as superficial harm to the head, perhaps like a scalp wound, in contrast to actual insult to the brain. To counter the implication that a head injury was insignificant, the term "brain injured" began to be used. Still, "brain injured" had a pejorative connotation. The phrase "survivor of a brain injury," or in common usage "survivor," then replaced "brain injured" to create the image of a person who has stature on par with that of therapists, insurers, families, etc. In this book, readers will note the use of the term "survivor" in the original definition of the neuropsychosocial environment from 1996. Persons with brain injury and professionals felt that this term provided recognition in a positive fashion of the person, while attending to the seriousness of their injury.

Nevertheless, the term "survivor" still suggests that the most important aspect of a person is the injury. Most recently, survivors have begun proposing the expression "person with brain injury." This phrase emphasizes that someone with a brain injury is a person first. It simultaneously addresses the idea that brain injury is the most serious of all injuries by not hiding behind less direct terms. The author believes that it is important to support the efforts of persons with brain injury to gain recognition of the fact that while their injuries ought not be minimized, they should not lose their humanity in the eyes of other people by being thought of as only their brain injury.

After all, therapists are not their jobs, but rather persons who provide care. People who lose sight of this are quickly depressed when they lose their jobs, having confused their roles as workers with their souls as people. Parents and spouses are not their roles, but people who have children or husbands and wives. Persons with brain injury are more than just brain injuries; they are people. The author believes that readers of this book will form a better, more appropriate impression of persons with brain injury through the use of this term.

In this book the term "therapist" is all-inclusive. It encompasses all disciplines including nurses, psychologists, neuropsychologists, physicians, case managers, behavioral technicians, behavioral analysts, psychology technicians, occupational therapists, physical therapists, speech language pathologists, recreational therapists, music therapists, chaplains, dieticians, group home staff, etc. In the approach this book presents, everyone who interacts with persons with brain injury creates the therapeutic environment. In regard to family members, they are identified specifically as family members when their unique role as a relative is pertinent, but otherwise the treatment procedure this book describes recognizes the importance of the therapeutic impact of family members and in that sense they are therapists, too.

Chapter 6 intentionally departs from this convention for the purposes of clarity. It uses "physician" in the unique role of writer of medication prescriptions and diagnostician of medical complications. Nevertheless, despite the unique role physicians have in respect to medications, they remain therapists in the neuropsychosocial approach. Everyone in contact with persons with brain injury is an important therapeutic component of the environment. Moreover, although this chapter uses the term physician, all therapists should take note of the information in this chapter regarding medication management. Just as physicians must appreciate behavioral interventions, so too must other therapists have knowledge of the hurdles physicians face in medication management, as well as the possibilities and limitations of medications. Also, therapists should be able to assist with the observation of symptoms and responses to medications and they will perform these tasks better with improved knowledge of medications.

A Special Note to Persons with Brain Injury

You may find that this book spends a great deal of time explaining the hurdles that some of you encounter because of your injury. This is intentional. Too often, the author sees persons with brain injury fall short of their potential because therapists fail to understand the problems with which persons with brain injury struggle. This is particularly true when the problem is behavioral dyscontrol. Unless they appreciate the difficulties each person faces, therapists cannot help individuals build on their strengths. Please do not be offended. I believe that even those persons with brain injury who have severe behavioral dyscontrol problems can achieve great things if therapists understand the root causes of dyscontrol.

It is my belief that there are two great challenges that therapists encounter when assisting persons with brain injury who exhibit behavioral dyscontrol. First, therapists must understand the problems causing the behavioral dyscontrol sufficiently. Second, therapists must innovate in designing treatment. This book, then, intends to educate therapists about behavioral dyscontrol and to encourage innovation. But, education cannot take place without examination of what is sometimes the unfortunate reality of severe behavioral dyscontrol.

Therefore, this book may shock many persons with brain injury and their advocates in its description of the behavioral problems of some persons with brain injury. It may be difficult for many persons with brain injury to conceive of their peers as doing the things that this book discusses. However, the descriptions contained in this book are not those of the author's wild imaginings, but are of the type that I have encountered in my clinical work.

I believe that unless we all openly acknowledge the behavior of this subset of persons with brain injury, we cannot help them reach their maximum potential. Still, the level of achievement for some persons with brain injury who exhibit severe behavioral dyscontrol may be less than what they, their therapists, their families, or other persons with brain injury would ideally hope to see happen. It is unfortunate, but true, that everyone working with persons with brain injury who demonstrate severe behavioral dyscontrol eventually faces the limitations imposed by each person's brain injury. Yet, despite the focus in this book on severe behavioral dyscontrol, persons with brain injury who read this book should know that the author realizes that not all persons with brain injury have behavioral problems. Moreover, the author recognizes that if persons with brain injury have behavioral problems these problems are usually not severe in nature.

This book is designed to help therapists serve persons with brain injury for whom everything else has failed. It intends to encourage therapists to fully address behavioral dyscontrol, even when it is emotionally hard for therapists to do so. Therapists wrestle every day with trying to help persons with brain injury who exhibit behavioral dyscontrol to have as few limitations as possible. Persons with brain injury should know that when restrictions remain, even after treatment for severe behavioral dyscontrol, it is emotionally difficult for therapists. However, the author believes that this book carries a very positive message amidst all the discussion about problems: even persons with brain injury who have severe behavioral problems can achieve amazing things. The author has been fortunate to see miracles happen for people who would otherwise be consigned to state hospitals or prisons. I have seen very dangerous people turn their lives around. I consider myself very lucky to have had the opportunity to help them. As for the majority of persons with brain injury, many of whom I count as some of the most dedicated, enjoyable, and wisest people I know, your support is invaluable. Thank you.

This Book and Prevention of Brain Injury

A word about prevention is appropriate. Prevention of brain injuries could eliminate all the problems that this book addresses. I have been struck by the impact of prevention efforts as illustrated in the following two anecdotes. First, when my niece got her first tricycle several years ago she immediately said, "Where is my helmet?" Second, when my then 10-year-old nephew found out that I was writing this book he asked me for the very first copy. Why? He wanted to take it to school to show his friends who do not wear bicycle helmets. If these children are astute enough to have learned about prevention of brain injury from educational campaigns and parental instruction, imagine what could be accomplished if adults were as smart about protecting other children and themselves from potential brain injuries.

So, I ponder the question, for example, of why parents insist that their children wear elbow and knee pads when rollerskating, but not helmets. Why do we see unhelmeted parents riding bicycles next to their helmeted child? Why do we see parents not wearing their seatbelts, but placing their children in car seats? It is as if these parents decided that a broken bone is more worrisome than a damaged brain or that children with brain injuries would be a tragedy, but these same children "losing" their parents to an avoidable brain injury would be less of a tragedy. Perhaps this book can serve as a warning to all adults about the consequences of brain injury and heighten their awareness of the need for prevention. After all, the best treatment for brain injury is prevention.

Notice

It is essential that readers of this book rely on their own judgment when dealing with persons with brain injury. They must do so with knowledge of the individual needs of the persons they wish to help and they must assume ultimate responsibility for their decisions, including behavioral and pharmacological judgments. This is particularly so when they address behavioral dyscontrol. Providing assistance to persons with brain injury who may exhibit behavioral dyscontrol entails risk of harm to therapists, others, and persons with brain injury. Nothing in this book removes that risk. It is the sole responsibility of the readers of this book to determine whether and how to apply the information this book contains. In addition, no single reference should serve as an exclusive source of information regarding brain injury behavioral or pharmacological interventions. Readers are advised to consult multiple sources of information (e.g., medication manufacturer's product information) before proceeding.

The clinical examples in this book reflect composite pictures of clinical situations. They draw upon an aggregate accumulation of clinical experience. Readers should not be misled to think that examples are actual people just because of similarities between examples and their own experiences. Similarities that appear may be indicative of the commonality of human behavior after brain injury. Nevertheless, readers must take responsibility to determine in what manner they choose to apply information from the clinical examples.

The author and contributors do not assume any liability for any harm, injury, or property damage stemming from this book.

chapter one

The neuropsychosocial approach

Introduction

Severe behavioral problems after acquired brain injury can challenge the therapeutic skills of even experienced professional care providers. Too often, extreme behavioral dysfunction perplexes therapists, leading to treatment failure. Traditional behavioral treatment strategies often fail to successfully address severe behavioral difficulties in the brain injury population; however, an innovative treatment approach can overcome even severe behavioral problems.

Brain injury may be acquired in a multitude of ways. The most common include traumatic events, such as motor vehicle crashes, sports injuries, falls, and assaults.[1] Gunshot injuries are also a frequent cause of traumatic brain injury. In children, shaken baby episodes may result in brain injury.[2] Lack of oxygen to the brain from a near-drowning episode, carbon monoxide exposure (from sources such as heater malfunction in ice houses used for winter fishing, or suicide attempt by automobile engine fume exposure), breathing cessation post motor vehicle crash, suicide attempt by hanging, heart attack sequelae, untoward surgical events, cerebrovascular accidents, brain tumors, and drug overdose can all cause brain injury. Another source of brain injury is toxic chemical exposure.[3] Finally, brain infection can lead to brain injury. Hence, the term "acquired brain injury" subsumes traumatic brain injury, anoxia, stroke, tumor, drug effects, and infection.

Other conditions that involve altered brain function include degenerative diseases such as Alzheimer's disease, multiple sclerosis, Parkinson's disease, and Pick's disease. Further causes of damage to the brain include congenital factors, birth trauma, or even pre-birth events — fetal alcohol or cocaine exposure. Mental retardation involves cognitive sequelae of altered brain function. However, while the treatment approach proposed here may be of benefit to these populations, the primary intent of this book is to address the treatment challenges that people with acquired brain injury present to families and professionals.

The number of brain injuries in the United States is staggering. Hospital emergency departments treat and release one million people each year for brain injury,[4] and many more people with brain injuries never seek care. The number of people needing care in hospitals and thereafter is large.[5] Approximately 230,000 Americans are hospitalized each year due to traumatic brain injury. If even a small percentage of persons with brain injury experience behavioral problems, providers, families, friends, employers, and society face a daunting challenge. Furthermore, many persons with brain injury are young at onset. Hence, left untreated, behavioral dysfunction will exhibit itself for decades.

The National Institutes of Health Rehabilitation of Persons with Traumatic Brain Injury Consensus Statement describes the annual cost of acute care and rehabilitation for new cases of traumatic brain injury as $9 to $10 billion, with the average lifetime cost of care after severe injury as $600,000 to $1,875,000 per person.[1] These enormous costs are an underestimate of overall costs because they fail to incorporate the economic impact of lost earnings, social services utilization, and lost economic contribution from family members. People with brain injury who exhibit severe dyscontrol are likely at the high end of the spectrum in regard to cost.

While severe behavioral problems are uncommon when one considers all persons with brain injury,[6] for those who experience dyscontrol the consequences are significant. Such behavior causes significant disruption for persons with brain injury and the people who come into contact with them. Extreme behavior demands attention.

Severe behavioral dyscontrol after acquired brain injury takes many forms. Persons with brain injury may threaten to harm themselves or other people. They may verbalize an intent to destroy property. They may engage in self-injurious behavior, hurt others, or aggress against objects. They may threaten to run away, or may actually elope. They may put themselves at risk for being taken advantage of by other people.

There are many ways to threaten to or actually hurt oneself. Persons with brain injury may self-mutilate by poking themselves with pins, pens or pencils, forks, or jewelry, or by scratching themselves with paper clips, notebook binders, bed frame edges, doorframes, fingernails, or any surface with a corner or edge. They may use a knife to cut themselves. They may burn themselves with matches, cigarettes, or stove burners; they may bang their heads against walls, floors, or objects. Persons with brain injury are at higher risk than the general population for the most destructive type of self-injurious behavior: suicide attempt.[7,8] An unsuccessful suicide attempt can worsen brain injury: an unsuccessful gunshot wound, hanging, or carbon monoxide exposure most certainly will aggravate brain damage already present.

Persons with brain injury may also direct aggression against other people. They may grab, pull, pinch, or twist. They can come up from behind and attempt to choke someone or put a knee into someone's back. They may grasp one's clothing and pull. A man's necktie is a particularly dangerous target, as it is essentially a slipknot or noose around the wearer's neck. Long hair also makes a tempting target. Earrings are another dangerous item that can easily be pulled, sometimes resulting in ripping of the ear lobe.

More direct forms of assault also take place. Hitting and kicking are the most common, though one may also encounter head butting. Sometimes the aggression represents indiscriminate lashing out, but at other times there is a marked intention to do bodily damage to another person. Persons with brain injury may spit, which can be particularly harmful if aimed at someone's eyes. Infrequently, a person with brain injury may propel other bodily fluids at another individual as well.

A frequent form of aggressive behavior is throwing things. The item thrown can range from ineffectual (crumpled up paper or clothes) to dangerous (a kitchen utensil, knife, or chair). A table can be flipped over towards another person, as can a bed. Unlikely objects can be turned into weapons. A notebook can be broken apart and a weapon created from the metal binder. A window can be broken and the sharp pieces used for weapons. Individuals can rip apart bathroom fixtures, making a weapon from faucet handles. Others may avail themselves of weapons which do not "require assembly," such as guns or knives.

In addition to the creation of weapons, persons with brain injury may engage in property destruction. They may punch holes in walls or damage appliances. A frequent target appears to be the telephone, when the person becomes angry during a phone conversation. Frustration during automobile rides leads to wear on automobile interiors. A person may set fire to objects, furniture, or a building in an expression of anger.

There are additional types of behavioral dysfunction which may be more subtle, but are disruptive nonetheless. Persons with brain injury may demonstrate poor safety decisions. They may persist in transferring from a wheelchair to a chair unassisted when they lack sufficient skill to do so, risking a fall. They may insist on driving before their therapists clear them to do so.

Persons with brain injury can become demanding or manipulative. They may pester with continual requests or pit one therapist against another. Noncompliance may be a problem — they may refuse treatment or medications, or they may use noncompliance as a bargaining tactic.

Social inappropriateness is a frequent problem. Persons with brain injury may have poor social skills. They may disregard or be unaware of social boundaries and appropriate behavior. They may make comments that are offensive to others or invade other people's personal space. Sexual inappropriateness may also cause problems, as they can become too forward or target the wrong person. Sexual assault is possible. In contrast to this type of behavior, some persons with brain injury become isolated and socially withdrawn. They may refuse to leave their rooms, as the world may seem overwhelming. Because their attempts at interaction are ineffective and cognitive deficits lead to mistakes, they feel that isolation is safer.

The cognitive deficits of persons with brain injury can become a behavioral problem, too. "Innocent" behavioral dyscontrol can result from cognitive dysfunction. Individuals may be confused or disoriented. Many persons with brain injury show an unawareness of their deficits. Some may experience delusions or hallucinations. Somatic complaints can arise out of proportion to physical health condition. Persistent somatic complaints can sometimes dominate all discourse with persons with brain injury. Obsessiveness may be displayed in the form of theft or hoarding of food or objects: pencils, crayons, and straws are commonly hoarded objects in hospitals.

Finally, elopement is a serious problem. Some persons with brain injury may run away, often with nowhere to go. Those with significant cognitive impairment may just wander away. Some persons with brain injury get lost. Some may put themselves in vulnerable positions, in which they can be emotionally exploited and abused. Persons with brain injury may be at risk for physical assault, theft, and rape.

The array of ways in which persons with brain injury exhibit dyscontrol is endless. Treatment procedures have traditionally been unable to successfully address the wide range of behavioral dysfunction, particularly when the behaviors are severe.

Alternatives to treatment

The social penalty of severe behavior left untreated is harsh. The social service or health care system may lock away persons with brain injury in state hospitals.[9] Institutionalization of this type can be expensive, and appropriate treatment may be lacking. Although therapists may develop appropriate treatment programs in some institutions, many persons with brain injury languish untreated or inappropriately diagnosed. Trends for deinstitutionalization are encouraging only insofar as government allocates sufficient funds for alternative, correctly designed treatment programs. Still, treatment for truly severe behavioral dyscontrol may require temporary, but perhaps extended removal from the environment to ensure the safety of persons with brain injury and that of others. Regardless, it is easier to close institutions than to guarantee an adequate, permanent funding stream for smaller and more diverse service vendors scattered across a geographic region. Furthermore, such smaller providers of deinstitutionalized care lack the time, political resources, and knowledge to successfully lobby for adequate funding as large institutions do. Hence, when the social service or health care system places persons with brain injuries in state institutions without correct diagnoses and available, appropriate treatment, or removes them from institutions without care and support commensurate with their severe behavioral dyscontrol, a successful long term outcome is highly unlikely. Parenthetically, persons with mental illness also face deinstitutionalization without adequate alternative services.[10]

The social penalty of untreated or mistreated severe behavioral dyscontrol after acquired brain injury may include incarceration by the criminal justice system. In fact, violence following a number of organic syndromes can lead to incarceration.[11] Unfortunately, the authorities imposing incarceration may either be unaware of or not appreciate the etiological factor of brain injury as a contributing factor or primary cause of the offending behavior.[12] Education regarding brain injury is lacking among health care providers. To suppose that it is greater among criminal justice workers is foolhardy.

Once a person with brain injury is incarcerated, the opportunity for treatment to ameliorate the behavioral dyscontrol is nil. Of course, the behavior may be suppressed in prison due to fear or lack of opportunity, as the person is in a cell under observation by armed guards. This is not treatment, and it will not generalize to the real world if brain injury was an important causal factor leading to the crime and incarceration. Punishment and fear can suppress behavior, but, as has been known for along time,[13] they do not teach alternative behaviors that are necessary to support generalization across settings or maintenance over time. As will be seen shortly, contingencies often fail as an intervention strategy for severe behavioral dyscontrol after acquired brain injury, even when therapists apply them in a more therapeutic, sophisticated manner than do jailers or prison guards

Incarceration in prison may worsen behavioral dyscontrol. This venue presents unintended instruction in anti-social values and modeling of violence as a coping strategy. Thus, society is left with incarceration as a poor intervention strategy and one more likely to increase behavioral dyscontrol after acquired brain injury than to cure it.

Persons with brain injury also run the risk of falling through the cracks in the social service system, and receiving no attention. With behavioral dyscontrol as a symptom, receiving no attention is an infrequent occurrence, but it can happen. Persons with brain injury often find encounters with social service systems and program funding sources to be perplexing and incomprehensible, as do many professionals! Unable to avail themselves of the resources that do exist, they become invisible. Some live on the streets or in shelters, and with their cognitive and emotional limitations leading to a lack of inhibition they are vulnerable to abuse or further brain injury from assault or substance abuse.

Professionals must address behavioral problems. There is no choice. The available options of institutionalization, incarceration, or invisibility are unacceptable for an enlightened society. Unlike many other health conditions, perhaps congenital in nature, with symptoms that appear before one is of an age to vote on taxes which will pay for health care services, or which one might avoid with a healthy diet and lifestyle, we are all only one drunk driver away from needing appropriate brain injury treatment. Hence, the development of treatment services for behavioral dyscontrol after brain injury should be encouraged by all members of society to ensure adequate care for citizens who may suffer brain injury in the future.

If persons with brain injury persist in behavior that defeats the application of cognitive or emotional advances, the treatment of their other brain injury symptoms is pointless. Persons with brain injury with good behavioral control who achieve emotional adjustment can deal with cognitive deficits. Persons with brain injury with good behavioral control and who compensate for cognitive deficits can seek emotional adjustment. However, no one will tolerate persons with brain injury who demonstrate adequate emotional adjustment and satisfactory compensation for cognitive deficits but physically assault someone who irritates them. Behavioral control is essential to reintegrate back into society.[14]

Unfortunately, while there have been advances in medical care for brain injury, there has not been a parallel advance in addressing extreme behavioral problems. Medical advances include better emergency rescue teams and paramedic response services, emergency rooms, neurosurgery, intensive care units, and acute rehabilitation. Specialty services now include brain injury chemical dependence treatment centers, brain injury pre-vocational and vocational programs, and brain injury residential group homes. Programs address insight and denial, and work on social skills and relationships. There are even services to evaluate driving skills after acquired brain injury. However, all of these are out of reach for those individuals whose behavior is too dysfunctional. Yet, therapists often find that behavioral problems are the most difficult to treat.[15]

Traditional treatment model for behavioral dyscontrol after brain injury

The most common treatment model for behavioral dyscontrol after brain injury consists of psychotherapy and medication, supplemented by a social support system to maintain appropriate behavior. Psychiatric hospitalization acts as a backup for peak behavioral crises. This model bears examination, since it is notoriously unsuccessful for the management of extreme behavior after brain injury. Traditional psychotherapy and medication management fail to achieve sufficient behavior change, the social support is inadequate in maintaining change, and psychiatric hospitalizations cannot stem the tide of behavioral crises.

Psychotherapeutic approaches

Close examination shows why this intervention paradigm fails. Psychotherapy traditionally consists of three main approaches: insight-oriented treatment, contingency management, and skill-building therapy. Most approaches to behavioral dyscontrol suggest the use of these methods.[16] However, each method has its drawbacks when the therapist applies it to cases of severe behavioral dyscontrol after acquired brain injury (see Table 1.1).

Insight-oriented approach

Insight-oriented treatment is based on the supposition that how clients think, and how they perceive people and events, dictates their behavior.

Table 1.1 Traditional Interventions

Insight-Oriented Approach		
Technique	**Theory**	**Issues**
Provide information	Information alters thinking and thinking alters behavior	Cannot express thinking Thinking does not alter due to cognitive deficits Alteration in thinking does not alter behavior

Contingency Management		
Technique	**Theory**	**Issues**
Manipulate consequences	Behavior alters due to consequences	Forget behavior Forget consequences Rebel against consequences Not act in own long term interest

Skill Building		
Technique	**Theory**	**Issues**
Teach new skills	New skills replace less effective behaviors	Cannot learn new skill Perseverates on old behavior Forgets to do new skill Distorts new skill

Hence, treatment focuses on the idea that via the provision of information, clients will change their way of thinking about themselves, others, and the world. Therapists pass information to their clients through direct statements or leading questions. Thus, therapists directly or indirectly — depending on the therapist's theoretical stance — assist clients in gaining a new viewpoint. The premise is that armed with the new perceptions and insights, clients will change their behavior. However, many persons with severe brain injury have difficulty forming a cogent world view. Their perspective can be inconsistent or disorganized. Even if they do have a consistent conceptual perspective on people and events, they may be unable to reliably express it. So many persons with severe behavioral dyscontrol after acquired brain injury struggle to merely get through the day that when asked about values and beliefs, they cannot answer, as their energies are focused more on survival than on reflection.

Cognitive deficits can lead to additional barriers to behavior change through insight-oriented approaches. Perseveration can lead to an inability to shift thoughts, perceptions, or attitudes. New insights are useless if the person with traumatic brain injury cannot adopt them because of the cognitive rigidity caused by organic damage. The person with a traumatic brain injury may relapse to ingrained dysfunctional pre-treatment beliefs. Some people with traumatic brain injury are unable to adopt alternative concepts because they cannot surmount the hurdles involved in perceiving the world from another person's perspective — a very complicated, high level cognitive task.

To adopt an alternative world view first requires people to understand their own views of other people, events, and the world, and then grasp the viewpoint of someone else. This includes appreciation of the values, both subtle and obvious, of the other person as well as how the other person applies those values and judgments to specific instances. Next, people need to suppress their own viewpoints. This means they must ignore their own value structures. This is difficult because values are often at the core of belief systems, and people learn them at a young age. Next, people have to examine their response to a particular event while they adopt the other person's perspective. Finally, to complete their understanding of some else's alternative viewpoint, they must compare how they felt about an event while trying on someone else's values with how they felt about the event while applying their original value system. In lay terms, this is cognitively "walking a mile in someone else's shoes." This is a difficult task for many uninjured people, and it can be nearly impossible for a person with brain injury. The number of steps involved and the cognitive sophistication entailed can be insurmountable for many persons with brain injury.

Even if persons with brain injury are able to change their viewpoint, perspectives, and perhaps values, behavioral change may still elude them. At the moment of behavioral dyscontrol — when irritated, aroused, and ready to physically strike out or elope — the link between world conceptualization and emotional drive state is too tenuous, because of organic brain disruption, to inhibit a behavioral explosion. An agreement not to hit someone — or even "contracting" to not do so — may have little effect when the person with severe dyscontrol problems becomes agitated.

Contingency management

The foundation of consequence utilization is the principle that clients will change their behavior in response to the result of that behavior. The task of the therapist is to manipulate contingencies — advisably by way of reinforcement rather than punishment — to change behavior. Reinforcement tends to facilitate more permanent change, while avoiding the ethical concerns that punishment engenders. In response to these contingencies, clients alter their behavior to achieve positive outcomes.

Persons with brain injury who exhibit severe behavioral dyscontrol frequently have cognitive deficits that greatly hinder the therapeutic application of contingency management techniques. When therapists apply consequences, persons with brain injury have often forgotten what behavior they performed that led to the consequence, because of organically based memory deficits. Shortly after the event they may actually deny, even with reminding, ever having carried out such behavior, due to either psychological denial or anosognosia.

In addition to having memory deficits which impact upon recall of a behavior, persons with brain injury may have forgotten about a previous consequence when a situation arises in which they can either repeat the behavior or choose an alternative action. Hence, the inappropriate behavior reoccurs. There may be little or no awareness that they have demonstrated the same or similar behavior in the past with resultant consequences. Forgotten consequences have no power to modulate future behavior.

Persons with brain injury who have sufficient memory ability to recall their behavior and its resultant consequences tend to rebel against the application of contingency management. Despite living in a society that readily accepts the universal contingency reward of money, all people dislike the notion that someone might otherwise attempt to control their behavior through the direct application of a reward system. Persons with brain injury are no different from the general citizenry in this regard.

Adults with brain injury who recollect their premorbid lives of independence resent the implied removal of their empowerment by a contingency management system. Therapists who administer contingency management systems implicitly challenge the person's sense of self-esteem when the therapists manipulate contingencies as one might do with a child.[17] This resentment may manifest itself even as the person with brain injury acknowledges that the behavior is out of control.

Since persons with brain injury can demonstrate behavioral dyscontrol of truly dangerous proportions to themselves and others, the addition of resentfulness in response to contingency management can exacerbate the situation. Therapists can be confronted by a greater degree of risk than they can outlast, waiting for consequences to impact behavior over multiple episodes of severe aggression. The rebound effect often seen after the initiation of contingency management, in which behavior worsens in the short run, is too severe in an adult otherwise deemed dangerous before the imposition of consequence manipulation.

Persons with brain injury may fail to act in their own long-term self-interest. Their brain injury may lead them to respond to internal drives separate from thoughtful reflection and rational judgment in a cost–benefit analysis. The immediate short-term removal of an irritation may be more worthwhile than any benefit therapists can provide. Social or long-term personal considerations become irrelevant, or at least less of a consideration. Sometimes no therapist-devised consequence matches the unadulterated emotional release of hitting someone. The repercussions do not matter. In such instances severe consequences might (or still might not) derail aggression, assuming that previous behavioral episodes and their consequences are available in the person's memory, but this type of consequence (e.g., food contingent on behavior) is unethical.

Skill-building treatment

The foundation of skill-building approaches is that when given two or more alternative behaviors to use in response to a problem, people will select the most efficacious choice. The therapist instructs the client in a skill to employ in place of previous dysfunctional behavior. The therapist teaches the client the skill so that there is an understanding about when and how to use it. It is assumed that due to enlightened self-interest, people will utilize the best skill option available to them to accomplish their goal or to solve a problem.

Persons with brain injury, however, can have extraordinary difficulty trying to learn a new skill. Cognitive processing deficits greatly interfere with skill acquisition. Attentional problems as well as learning and memory weakness hinder instruction. Moreover, concept formation limitations mean many persons with brain injury fail to grasp the nuances of a skill and the necessary technique to implement it.

Cognitive deficits also affect practice of a new skill. Persons with brain injury can be insensitive to feedback. They may omit suggestions from the therapist about adaptations to and improvement in their technique. When they initially try a new skill, if they achieve a less positive outcome than they expected, they might abandon the effort altogether.

Avoidance of behavioral dysfunction requires skill application at the moment that emotional irritability, agitation, and arousal are building. The very emotional turmoil that the therapist intends the skill to prevent from leading to behavioral dyscontrol hinders the successful application of the skill. People do not perform at their best when they are emotionally distraught. It is unreasonable to expect persons with brain injury to do better, and there are obvious cognitive and emotional reasons to expect poorer performance.

Cognitive problems may also cause persons with brain injury to lack success when it is time to apply a new skill. They may be able to grasp the purpose of a skill, learn the skill, incorporate adaptations, continue to practice in the face of preliminary failures, and finally acquire expertise, but may then be unable to implement it expeditiously when they need it the most. Sometimes they may be too late in the sequence of real world events to try the skill. Due to slowed cognitive processing speed or impairments in reasoning abilities, the new skill may come to mind after the opportunity to try it has passed. Memory deficits may cause them to forget to employ the new skill at all. Also, rigidity in cognitive processing may cause them to relapse, perseverating on a previous behavior regardless of their recall of the new technique.

For those persons with brain injury who can overcome the emotional distress of the moment and remember to use the new skill, the final challenge is to correctly implement the skill. Therapists often observe distorted versions of a new skill, in contrast to the purer form the person with brain injury demonstrated during skill instruction. Getting it all right in order to be truly useful is difficult. Poorly implemented skills are usually ineffective and cause frustration, decreasing the probability that the person will attempt these alternative behaviors again. This initiates a self-fulfilling cycle of futility, with resistance to experimenting with new skills in the future.

Persistence of the traditional psychotherapeutic model

Many therapists and programs continue to rely on this interventional model, which persists in part because of the nature of our treatment system. Therapists learn insight-oriented, contingency management, and skill-building procedures in classes, practica, and internships during professional training. These approaches become comfortable and familiar. Their comfort with these interventions reflects their preconceived notions of the services that they would be taught to provide during training to be therapists. Moreover, once in practice, therapists can take comfort in the certainty that they have faithfully applied their training, conforming to the accepted model of treatment, if treatment should fail. They did as they were trained, and success or failure is the client's responsibility.

When these strategies are applied in individual interaction with the person who seeks help, there exist definable, discrete moments of therapeutic interaction during which therapists are clearly providing therapy. This model fits the conventional notion for persons with brain injury of being "in" therapy, and for therapists, of "doing" therapy: there are therapy sessions. This is helpful in the implementation of traditional therapy, because typically clients' expectations and a "shared world view" about the role of the therapist, what constitutes therapy, and the therapist's armamentarium are crucial factors in reaching therapeutic success.[18]

With regard to reimbursement, there are clear, well established, firmly standardized,[19] and often rigid mechanisms for reimbursement for traditional treatment. Third party reimbursement sources are most receptive to discretely occurring treatment events, so one can bill for treatment sessions. Third party insurers often will not reimburse therapists or programs for truly therapeutic activities that may be more crucial to the treatment outcome than the "session" components of an overall treatment program. In addition, health care documentation and quality assurance compliance assessment prefer the discrete session model.

Medication management

Medication management is another element of the traditional approach to behavioral dyscontrol after brain injury. Medication management and the psychotherapeutic approaches of insight, skill building, and contingency management commonly work together. However, medication management for severe behavioral dyscontrol after brain injury gives rise to a host of problems. A full delineation of these issues and discussion of how professionals can address these concerns in order to successfully use medications for behavioral dyscontrol can be found in Chapter 6. Nevertheless, a preliminary examination of these challenges will highlight the shortcomings of trying to rely on this traditional approach.

Professionals attempting medication management often adjust medication treatment inadequately for the presence of brain injury. Hence, medications may be used to sedate persons with brain injury, thereby controlling behavior, but at the cost of cognitive function. Also, concurrent medical problems common to brain injury (seizures, for example) may complicate the utilization of psychotherapeutic medication in the brain injury population.

Many persons with brain injury can demonstrate a clearing of behavioral dyscontrol with discontinuation of many of the medications that were originally prescribed to help control their behavior. Most treatment settings, however, are hesitant to attempt lowering or removal of medication, since medication weaning can be a lengthy process and there may be escalation of behavioral dyscontrol during medication decrease.

Medication management is made even more difficult by the ever-changing frequency, intensity, and type of behavioral dyscontrol persons with brain injury may exhibit. Early in recovery their status is evolving. As time passes and they complete initial recovery, other issues arise. Factors such as aging or hormonal changes can play a role in the expression of behavioral dyscontrol. Changes in the environment can trigger stress. Hence, medication management is often like trying to hit a moving target of behavioral dyscontrol. Nevertheless, medication management, used correctly, can be very helpful in achieving behavioral control and stability, as will be seen in Chapter 6.

Support systems

A linchpin of the traditional treatment model is the non-institutional, natural, social support system of persons with brain injury. This social support network includes families, friends, and employers, among others, who may have an interest in the success of the person with brain injury. This support system facilitates generalization across settings and maintenance over time of the treatment professionals provide. Independent from the philosophical orientation of traditional treatment and the constellation of medications a physician prescribes, the person with brain injury depends upon the assistance of the support system for ultimate success in the community.

Despite their importance, social support systems repeatedly fail to meet the needs of the person with brain injury. Family members burn out on having to continually address behavioral crises. They tire of being required to put their own emotional needs on hold, secondary to the needs of the person with brain injury, because family members cannot place the person's needs after their own without triggering behavioral dyscontrol. It is wearying to always come second.

Family members risk losing their own social outlets in their efforts to serve the needs of the person with brain injury. Families may experience stress and role changes.[20,21,22,23] The recreational and community activities of family members decrease as they devote more time to the person with brain injury. Friends can become distant, and family members feel isolated.

The health of family members can deteriorate. It is common for professionals to observe family members rapidly aging in appearance. A family member may look ten years older over the course of the first year of care. Family members may demonstrate significant fatigue. They may be sleeping poorly. They may have to forego vacations due to lack of reliable, cost-acceptable respite care that can handle episodes of behavioral dyscontrol. They may take the person with the brain injury along on vacation, only to find that it is more stressful to handle the behavioral outbursts in a vacation setting than in the familiar home setting with resources nearby. Therapists often see depression and hopelessness among family members.

The financial stability of family members can be at risk. They must sometimes decrease their work hours to provide care for the person with brain injury. Employment may be terminated as a result of excessive time off work or poor performance at work due to fatigue or distractibility. Financial instability and lost work are particularly devastating, since health costs to family members can escalate dramatically after brain injury. Moreover, persons with brain injury can cause expensive damage to property.

Finally, family members may have to withdraw as care providers due to safety concerns. The person with brain injury may physically threaten or assault them. Some persons with brain injury find children particularly irritating, as they can be noisy, demanding, and unpredictable. Such behaviors on the part of children may trigger behavioral dyscontrol by a person with brain injury, and children may be at risk.

Friends also may decrease their commitment to helping the person with brain injury over time. Friends move on; they may have new jobs or go to school. They establish new relationships. Perhaps they move to a more distant neighborhood or to a new city or state. They have children. While these events occur, the person with brain injury is frozen in time: not getting married, advancing in a career, or making new friends. In addition, because of behavioral dyscontrol episodes, friends exclude the person with brain injury from major events in their lives. Hence, the component of friendship based on shared, or at least similar, experiences is gone. The friendship becomes less tenable and dissolves. The former friends are no longer available as a piece of the social support system.

Employers may struggle to maintain a relationship with the person with brain injury. Many people after a brain injury are unable to return to their former jobs. Only employers with a true commitment to the person with brain injury provide or help find a suitable alternative position. Moreover, once episodes of behavioral dyscontrol take place, it is very rare for an employer to continue to employ the person with brain injury. After employment is terminated, employers rarely remain part of the social support system.

The inability of the social support network to adequately sustain a person with brain injury in the community is not surprising. It reflects society's lack of preparedness to respond to chronic illness in general, and dealing with episodes of behavioral dyscontrol may be the most difficult of all situations. People are taught directly or through modeling what society expects when someone is ill.

Society assigns everyone a role when an injury or illness occurs.[24] Imagine, for instance, someone breaks a leg. The health care worker is a compassionate person who has the time to take an interest in the injured individual beyond the diagnosis, and provides knowledgeable care, education, and case coordination. Classic television physicians such as Dr. Kildare, Marcus Welby, M.D., or Hawkeye Pierce come to mind. Family members put their lives on hold to help the hurt person. They take time off work. They drive the individual to appointments. They bring breakfast in bed. Insurance companies recognize the importance and appropriateness of treatment. They readily agree to immediate radiographic studies of the broken leg, as well as to subsequent serial studies. Authorization for outpatient procedures (e.g., setting the leg) or inpatient procedures (e.g., surgery) is easily forthcoming. Additional treatment, perhaps physical therapy, is routine. They authorize equipment needs, such as crutches or a wheelchair, quickly. Friends pitch in to help. Perhaps they bring over meals. In cold climates they may shovel snow off the injured person's driveway. Sympathy cards and flowers arrive at the home or hospital room of the hurt person. Many friends visit to offer condolences and support. Employers hold open the injured person's job. They may call, come to visit, or send a token of their concern. Injured people have a role, too. They take time off from work, rest, and follow the health care plan. Most importantly, they get better.

The understanding is that if the patient, health care provider, family, friends, and employer all follow their roles, the patient gets better and essentially everyone returns to their role of friend, employer, or family member just like before the injury. Society accepts that the injured person may have some slight residual problems, but none that would require any substantial adjustment or ongoing support.

When someone suffers an incurable injury, such as a brain injury, or has an incurable chronic disease (e.g., kidney difficulty necessitating ongoing dialysis, or disabling low back pain), the pact with society falls apart. People play their roles correctly, but the hurt person is not cured. Residual problems continue to impact family, friends, and employers who now do not know what to do, or are emotionally or financially unprepared. So, they burn out.

When the presenting health problem is merely medical in nature, it is very difficult on the social support system, but when it includes behavioral dyscontrol it is worse. People not only burn out; they actively seek to distance themselves from the dangerous person. The loss of social support compounds the potential devastation of the brain injury.

Psychiatric hospitalization

The treatment of last resort in the traditional model of care is psychiatric hospitalization. When all else fails in the care of an individual with a brain injury who exhibits ongoing behavioral dysfunction at a level others are unwilling to tolerate, the health care system offers hospitalization on a psychiatric unit. Unfortunately, traditional psychiatric hospitalization often proves fruitless for truly severe behavioral dyscontrol after a brain injury. In truth, even in cases of so-called mild brain injury the mental health system is naïve about brain injury symptomatology.[25]

As will be seen in Chapter 2, therapists must adjust treatment for persons with brain injury to account for cognitive deficits.[26] Hence, standard individual or group approaches, from all philosophical counseling models, test insufficient when therapists apply them to persons with brain injury. Moreover, beyond the concern of the applicability of counseling techniques to those persons with brain injury is the typical lack of knowledge that psychiatric unit therapists have about the challenges and issues persons with brain injury and their families face. Training for psychiatrists in the treatment of brain injury has historically been lacking.[27]

Persons with brain injury tend to reject treatment that lumps them in with other diagnostic categories, including mental illness, mental retardation, or developmental disability. The difficulties people with those diagnoses encounter may seem similar on the surface, but there are fundamental differences. Many people with brain injuries lived normal lives prior to onset. Their expectations were those of a "normal" person. Therapists must consider fundamentally different issues when they structure treatment for a person who, for example, has been developmentally delayed since childhood compared with, for example, a business executive who is the victim of a motor vehicle accident, though both might now exhibit superficially similar behavioral aggression. Life circumstances prior to brain injury onset make a difference.

The natural course of recovery for people with diagnoses from different diagnostic categories can show significant distinctions. In fact, the concept of "recovery" may apply poorly to certain diagnoses. Therapists who are unaware of the nature of acquired brain injury are likely to miss important factors crucial to successful treatment. Etiology makes a difference. Moreover, there are likely to be material, qualitative differences in the behavioral dyscontrol of persons with brain injury compared to other people. Chapter 4 will explore the phenomenology of behavioral dyscontrol. A therapist who lacks experience with persons with brain injury may miss or misunderstand variables that may greatly influence the efficaciousness of treatment. Qualitative factors make a difference.

Traditional psychiatric care includes administration and management of medications. As noted earlier, if medication is used, the organic changes induced by brain injury must be taken into consideration . Medication management for behavioral dyscontrol after acquired brain injury requires special understanding of the effects of various medications on persons with brain injury. Chapter 6 will review this in detail.

Finally, therapists providing traditional inpatient psychiatric care may encounter problems making appropriate discharge plans. Many traditional post-discharge resources are inappropriate for persons with brain injury. For example, chemical dependency programs that cater to a non-brain injury population may be inappropriate. The discharge planner must be familiar with specialized brain injury residential sites. The person with brain injury will need special support group services. Financial resource services are different for persons with brain injury. Specific knowledge about brain injury is necessary to conduct proficient discharge planning. Absent appropriate discharge planning with links to appropriate post-hospital resources and follow-up services, the result is a potential revolving door of psychiatric hospitalizations. Discharge planning makes a difference.

Summary

The traditional model of treatment fails persons with brain injury who exhibit severe behavioral dysfunction. This treatment model, consisting of insight-oriented therapy, contingency management, and skill-building psychotherapeutic approaches, is not sufficient to overcome the cognitive challenges that brain injury can impose. Medication management is difficult to conduct although, as will be seen, it can be quite effective when the physician adapts it to the challenges of brain injury. The social support network often disintegrates when its members confront a friend's or family member's chronic behavioral dysfunction after acquired brain injury. The safety net of traditional psychiatric hospitalization is fraught with pitfalls for persons with brain injury, raising serious doubts as to its applicability in these cases. A new approach is needed.

Neuropsychosocial approach

The traditional treatment model is designed to change persons with brain injury to fit the world. The world consists of a physical environment and interactions with people, and society expects its members — including persons with brain injury — to conform to its physical and social demands. Through insight-oriented, contingency management, and skill-building therapies supplemented by the administration of medications, the purpose of traditional intervention is to help persons with brain injury blend into the world.

Therapists rarely question this ingrained idea. Yet in other therapeutic endeavors, with other populations, therapists frequently profess a different goal. Therapists readily accept, for example, a treatment goal of being comfortable with oneself — "knowing who you are," self-actualization, or assertiveness about being at ease with one's unique attitudes and behaviors. The purpose of this type of treatment is personal comfort with one's self rather than fitting into the world. Nevertheless, when therapists address "unacceptable" behaviors by persons with brain injury, they apply a different philosophy: the person with brain injury must change to accommodate the world. O'Dowd provided seminal insights into the inappropriateness of this methodology.[28] He argued for an ecological approach in which therapists would go beyond traditional treatment to work not just *with* the environment or *in* the environment, but *on* the environment. For some time, therapists have taken an essentially environmental approach to address behavioral issues for persons with brain injury during the early stages of treatment.[29]

It is wonderful when persons with brain injury can change to conform to the world, if they wish to do so. Unfortunately, as previously discussed, too often persons with brain injury continue to exhibit behavioral dyscontrol, demonstrating an inability to adjust to the world despite the efforts of therapists through insight-oriented, contingency management, or skill-building therapies supplemented with medications.

This traditional treatment model fails because it espouses the wrong goal. The goal of treatment for a person with brain injury who fails to respond to traditional procedures should be to fit the world to the person with brain injury. The focus of intervention is on the world, not the person with brain injury.

Changing the world is the essence of the neuropsychosocial approach to intervention. The intent of this approach is to create around each person with brain injury a world in which that person can function well: a "neuropsychosocial environment." By making the philosophical conceptual shift to this approach, therapists can successfully manage disruptive behavior and in many cases eliminate it entirely.

Hence, the immediate goal of the neuropsychosocial approach is to create a neuropsychosocial environment. The neuropsychosocial environment is defined as follows:

> **The world experience created around survivors of organic impairment by people** and **physical space design**, which when correctly conceived and implemented, permits survivors to function with maximum cognitive, emotional, and behavioral success. It is the **culmination of understanding the interaction of survivors' neurological and neuropsychological assets and deficits** with the **social and psychological demands** of the environment to function in an acceptable societal manner. Knowledge of **how survivors experience the world — their phenomenology, gained from trained observation, cognitive assessment, and applied trials** — permits expert providers to develop a unique experience for each survivor. **Creation of an individualized neuropsychosocial environment** results in success beyond traditional psychotherapeutic or behavioral approaches: insight, contingency, or skill building therapies.[30]

A thorough understanding of the myriad treatment implications of this definition is critical for success when treating severe behavioral dyscontrol after acquired brain injury. Knowledge of what a neuropsychosocial environment is and how to create it will guide the methodologies that therapists require in conducting intervention.

A neuropsychosocial environment is an environment in which the person with brain injury can function well. If the person with brain injury is deficient in a skill which usually helps with behavioral control and the person cannot learn or perform it, then the neuropsychosocial environment of that person is one in which that skill is unnecessary. If the person with brain injury lacks insight regarding someone or something and that lack of insight would normally lead to behavioral dyscontrol, then the neuropsychosocial environment of that person is complete without requiring that insight for that person to act appropriately. If the person with brain injury responds poorly to contingencies and correct responses to those contingencies would typically facilitate behavioral control, then the neuropsychosocial environment of that person permits them to behave correctly without requiring response to those contingencies.

The neuropsychosocial environment is a world in which the deficits of the person with brain injury do not matter because those qualities are unnecessary for that person in that world to maintain behavioral control. For uninjured people, the world is full of challenges that can be stressful. However, most people, including most persons with brain injury, avoid severe loss of control when they face challenges to their conceptualizations and abilities. For a person with brain injury who exhibits severe loss of behavioral control and is unable to benefit from traditional treatment, the solution is to produce a world with only challenges that the person is equipped to handle.

It is alien to many lay people, as well as therapists, to contemplate a world where all of the demands the environment imposes on someone are exactly the demands the person is best able to handle. This would be a world where the demands are within one's abilities. This would be a world that should be as ideal as could be made for each person. This world would obviously be different for each person in order to fit each person's abilities and concepts. For people with brain injury who fail traditional treatment, creation of such a world, the neuropsychosocial environment, is a practical, very effective, innovative treatment.

The creation of a neuropsychosocial environment for each person with brain injury exhibiting severe behavioral dyscontrol may appear to be a daunting task. The hurdles therapists face to construct this world may seem insurmountable, but they are not. It is feasible and efficacious for a skilled therapist to produce an environment that dovetails with the needs of a person with brain injury who demonstrates severe behavioral dyscontrol.

It may seem that the creation of this ideal world would isolate the person with brain injury from the "real" world. This is not so. Rather, it allows these people to participate in the "real" world up to their abilities to do so, instead of placing them in a state hospital or prison. The neuropsychosocial environment changes the regular world only to the minimal degree necessary for the person to succeed. In practice, reasonable modifications may be required to ensure success. The challenge to the therapist is to correctly conceptualize the essential modifications and to coordinate consistent implementation, not engineer wholesale transformation.

"The world experience created...by people..."

To create the appropriate world experience for a person with brain injury, the therapist must begin with a consideration of the people with whom the person with the brain injury comes into contact. For most human beings, dealing with other people is the greatest challenge they confront. Hence, the strongest determinant of the nature of the world everyone faces is how the people they encounter behave. People create experiences for one another.

The therapist must be adept at having the people who populate the world of the person with brain injury act in a manner conducive to the maintenance of that person's behavioral control. For the therapist, this is an art based upon knowledge of the person's emotional and cognitive strengths and weaknesses.

It is a challenge for the therapist to appropriately constitute the world around the person with brain injury. Beyond knowledge of the person's abilities, it requires teamwork and political skill. Other people on the team —professionals, family members, friends, and employers — must receive education and skill training on how to behave. Everyone the person with brain injury encounters should be viewed as a potential therapist. This includes nurses, social workers, physicians, psychologists, occupational therapists, speech pathologists, physical therapists, recreational therapists, music therapists, dietitians, chaplains, administrators, housekeepers, transportation staff, academic tutors, residential workers, etc. There must be a commitment on the part of all of these individuals to invest their energy in the cause of the person with brain injury and to modify their behavior according to his or her needs. Pulling this together requires political astuteness on the part of the therapist. Therapists recruit the cooperation of others in contact with the person with the brain injury, and everyone must act in concert to provide the person with consistent experiences.

Everyone who interacts with a person with brain injury influences how the person perceives the world. They all constitute the environment of the person with brain injury.[31] No one is immune from affecting the person with brain injury, and therefore everyone is responsible for the occurrence of behavioral dyscontrol. In the neuropsychosocial approach, everyone involved must be aware of the kind of world the treatment team is attempting to create. If any one therapist on a team is out of step, then the experience of the person with brain injury changes. Inconsistency creates an experience of unpredictability and unreliability for the person with brain injury, which will not help with behavioral control. Some therapists believe that 95% of maladaptive behaviors can be accounted for by how therapists behave.[32]

Therapists who create a neuropsychosocial environment are part of the world of the person with brain injury. Therapists must consider themselves as a component helping to form this world. In many treatment programs, therapists may constitute the majority of the people the person with brain injury engages with during the day. Hence, it is absolutely essential that therapists recognize the contribution their own behavior makes in establishing the world that a person with brain injury experiences.[33]

The most powerful tool therapists possess is the ability to manipulate their own behavior and to guide the behavior of the people who inhabit the world of the person with brain injury. Therapists must intentionally manipulate how they and others present themselves to the person with brain injury to create a unique, appropriate experience for each person with brain injury in light of that person's behavioral dyscontrol. It is impossible for therapists to be too aware of the importance of their own behavior in forming the experiential world of the person with behavioral dyscontrol after acquired brain injury. People have the greatest stimulus value in each other's world; in treatment for behavioral dyscontrol, the significance of the therapist's behavior is the key to the treatment program.

In traditional treatment, therapists focus on the content of their therapeutic activities: ambulation in a hallway, utilization of a kitchen utensil, taking medications, or discussion of self-image. In the neuropsychosocial approach, while these may be necessary components of treatment, they are insufficient to gain control of severe behavioral dyscontrol. Every detail of an interaction with a person with brain injury determines the therapeutic impact on behavioral dyscontrol. Hence, therapists' contributions to behavioral control extend beyond accomplishment of the immediate task at hand. Therapists must broaden their conceptualization of their encounters with the person with brain injury. In regard to behavioral dyscontrol, the therapeutic experience of persons with brain injury consists of the culmination of all their experiences during the course of treatment.

In the neuropsychosocial approach, therapists focus on how they present themselves and what their impact is on persons with brain injury, more than on particular treatment tasks. Therapists must be cognizant of their word choice and tone, attitude, body language, appearance, affect, timing, etc. All of these elements constitute the experience of persons with brain injury. Process variables are as important as event variables. How something happens is as important as what happens. In the neuropsychosocial approach, treatment plans delineate how therapists will interact with persons with brain injury. Plans focus on procedures and methodologies that therapists and others will use to relate to the person. Hence, treatment plans address therapists' behavior.

Traditionally, when a person with brain injury shows dyscontrol, the locus of responsibility is the person with the brain injury. In the neuropsychosocial approach, therapists recognize that their own behavior may require adjustment to generate a world in which the person with brain injury can avoid dyscontrol. When a person with brain injury acts inappropriately, therapists working in a program espousing a neuropsychosocial approach ask what *they* can do differently. Therapists who adapt a neuropsychosocial approach must be self-assured and confident in their skills. The team members must be emotionally supportive of each other. When a therapist acknowledges that a different tactic than the one taken might have led to better behavioral control on the part of the person with brain injury, the team must be able to pull together to avoid the ineffective (and perhaps dangerous) strategy again without disintegrating into blame of the therapist whose tactic fell short. This is challenging given that the traditional tendency in such situations is to blame the shortcomings on the person with brain injury or for team members to blame each other. Neuropsychosocial treatment demands therapists who know that the focus of attention when a person with brain injury fails is going to be upon them, but who can avoid placing blame, support each other, and use the knowledge they gain from each interaction to fine-tune the environment, as reflected in their interpersonal interactions, to the abilities of the person with the brain injury. This can be emotionally draining. The need for team support cannot be minimized.

Incalculable personal variables are available to therapists to manipulate. No description can be all-inclusive. Table 1.2 lists sufficient variables to provide therapists with a reasonable start and an understanding of how broadly they can conceive the variables available for manipulation

"...and physical space design..."

In addition to manipulation of interpersonal factors, therapists can specify physical space variables to assist with behavioral control. Uninjured people respond to their physical environment, and so do persons with brain injury. Persons with brain injury who exhibit behavioral dyscontrol may be more sensitive and responsive to physical alteration in their environment than uninjured people. Their tolerance for change in their physical world is often poor; change can easily trigger behavioral dyscontrol. Adapting the physical world can prove to be more of a challenge to therapists than coordinating interpersonal dynamics.

People may be willing to alter their behavior, but (in part as a reflection, perhaps, of the importance to them of their own physical space design needs) they can be quite resistant to modifications in the physical environment to conform to the needs of a person with brain injury at the cost of their own physical space and environmental preferences. Consider, for example, the dance of accommodation that new roommates, housemates, or married couples engage in as they negotiate the pitfalls of living together. Fights over temperature, lighting, and furniture are so common as to be the standard fare of stand-up comedians. Everyone is familiar with disagreements about bedroom clutter and bathroom routines.

Imagine the behavioral dyscontrol that persons with brain injury may exhibit in response to a physical world they find emotionally stressful

Table 1.2 Presentation Variables for Therapists to Manipulate

Structural Factors
Time of day, frequency of meeting
Duration of meeting, group vs. individual
Presence of other therapists
Verbal Presentation
Voice: volume, pitch, speed, pauses
Language: vocabulary, sentence complexity
Verbal Content
Number of steps in train of logic, analogies
Degree of abstraction, number of topics
Humor, self-depreciation
Nonverbal Presentation
Gestures: type, speed
Touch: where, duration, type, firmness
Body Posture: forward/back, sit/stand, closeness, arms/legs crossed
Face: expressions, eye contact
Emotional tone
Dress: casual vs. formal
Writing: note-taking on pad of paper, writing on white board

and cognitively challenging. While uninjured persons may tolerate parts of their world being annoying if they can sometimes retreat to a space they prefer or can control, for persons with brain injury who exhibit severe behavioral dyscontrol, having a refuge may be insufficient. Their world may need to be more conducive to behavioral control across places and situations.

Hence, therapists must confront the challenge of physical environmental engineering in numerous locations inhabited by the person with brain injury. This can prove difficult, since each locale may have different detrimental stimuli. Therapists must mold these into a consistent pattern across locations.

Sometimes therapists accomplish alterations in the physical environment with negligible impact on other people who share that environment. At other times re-engineering is more significant, requiring therapists to demonstrate significant negotiation skills. Cost, too, can be an important consideration. Therapists need flexibility when they contemplate physical space changes. Much as a photographer must learn to "see" details and patterns in a picture that make it pleasing — beyond the observation of the lay person, unaware of the details, who appreciates a photograph as a whole — therapists must see all of the elements which constitute the physical environment, to make it "pleasing" in the sense of conducive to behavioral control for the person with brain injury. Of course, each person with brain injury who exhibits behavioral dyscontrol may require a physical space with different design elements.

Table 1.3 Physical Space Variables for Therapists to Manipulate

Room
Size, color, decoration style, single vs. shared
Bathroom private vs. shared, windows, TV/radio
Type and amount of furniture
Locks
Doors, windows, closets, bathrooms, furniture drawers
Kitchen drawers, refrigerator, supply cabinet, thermostat
Furniture
Chairs vs. couches, recliners, rockers
Heaviness of furniture
Common Areas
Size, access, carpet or tile markings delineating boundaries, presence of stairs, access outside
Comfort Factors
Lighting, temperature, noise

A comprehensive list of physical design elements available to therapists with their specifications is impossible. Table 1.3 suggests variables to consider and provides therapists with a place to start.

"... culmination of understanding the interaction of survivors' neurological and neuropsychological assets and deficits..."

Therapists must understand the organic damage and the subsequent neuropsychological functioning of a person with brain injury to correctly design a neuropsychosocial environment. Appreciation of neuropathology and its effect on cognitive abilities is the foundation of insight into the behavioral performance of persons with brain injury. Absent this knowledge, therapists will flounder in treatment. As will be seen in Chapter 2, determination of cognitive functioning and study of its implications for behavioral dyscontrol is prominent in the creation of a neuropsychosocial treatment plan.

To formulate a treatment plan, therapists must know the cognitive capabilities and limitations of the person with brain injury. The responses of persons with brain injury to other people and to their physical environment are based upon their cognitive functioning. Their perceptions about their world are a result of their cognitive processing. Therapists, using knowledge of cognitive functioning to create a neuropsychosocial environment in which people behave in a manner conducive to behavioral control on the part of the person with brain injury, are extending a principle applied in insight-oriented psychotherapy after milder cases of brain injury. In this approach, the therapist adapts communication style — choice of words, rate of speech, use of gestures, and memory aids — to meet the needs of the person with brain injury in counseling. Similarly, therapists who are used to altering physical space during counseling — placement of a desk, presence of a softer light, etc. — are familiar with altering client responses through physical space environmental manipulation. Application of this concept in cases of behavioral dyscontrol requires therapists to extend this practice to an arena outside the office and to consider more thoroughly the cognitive functioning of the person with brain injury. In Chapter 2, there will be an examination of various cognitive variables and their application to treatment considerations.

"... social and psychological demands..."

Emotions are commonly driven by the interaction of desires and opportunities or lack thereof. When people can achieve what they want, they experience positive emotions. When the world deprives people of the attainment of their desires, negative emotions result. The social and psychological limitations placed upon people by society can thwart wishes or allow attainment of goals, permitting satisfaction. Demands to behave in a socially acceptable fashion pressure people to conform to societal standards in order to be rewarded for reaching goals society finds acceptable.

Hence, the world experience of the person with brain injury is a function of the person's behavior and what society thinks about it. Behaviors occur in context. Society determines the context, defining whether behavior is good or bad, acceptable or not. The product of behavioral selections made contrary to societal norms is, at minimum, disapproval and, at the extreme, turmoil. Therefore, therapists must be attentive to the standards to which other people expect the person with brain injury to adhere.

Failure to conform arises, in part, from cognitive impairment. First, cognitive impairment can reduce awareness of societal standards. In such instances, persons with brain injury may be nonconformists unintentionally, and suffer the consequences without knowing why. Second, cognitive impairment can lead to an inability to adhere to normative social and psychological expectations even when persons with brain injury know the standards. Their cognitive dysfunction makes them unable to behave appropriately. Third, some persons with brain injury who demonstrate severe behavioral dyscontrol exhibit casual disregard of normative behavior. They may know what is appropriate but choose to act otherwise. However, they often lack full recognition of the consequences of their choices, having made their decisions due to poor cognitively-based processing and judgment. In any case, uninjured people tend to tolerate behavior that violates their social and psychological norms poorly.

Emotional impairment also imposes difficulties on conformity, exacerbating problems arising from cognitive impairment. Organic brain injury can cause direct disruption of emotional status due to brain changes, and indirect emotional distress as the person with brain injury reacts to the realities of life after a brain injury. Distorted emotional drives can produce inappropriate behavior. When the brain signals anxiety, fear, or sexual need inappropriate to the environmental context, persons with brain injury respond to their internally determined drive state, often stunning other people with the nature of their behavior. Interestingly, persons with brain injury who are able to later recall or reflect upon their own behavior may show disbelief and embarrassment in regard to their own actions.

Emotions arising from adjustment to disability can be almost as powerful as distorted emotional drives in the determination of behavioral dyscontrol. As discussed previously, the expectation of society for the patient's role sets standards that people with chronic conditions are often unable to meet and may, in fact, be unhealthy in the long run. Nevertheless, both the person with brain injury who premorbidly endorsed those societal norms, and society itself, expect adjustment to proceed in a mutually agreed-upon fashion. Strong emotions arise when the course of recovery and subsequent limitations for the person with brain injury fall short of normative expectations. Anger, depression, grief, mistrust, and denial are potent emotional forces that drive behavior.

Therapists can intervene to change the expectations that others impose on the person with brain injury in cases where cognitive compensation or improvement in emotional expressivity consistent with environmental context are unachievable. Therapists need to provide assistance to those in the environment of the person with brain injury to set expectations for cognitive and emotional functioning congruent with the person's ability.

Behavioral dyscontrol is a common outcome when persons with brain injury are unable to perform cognitively or emotionally in the manner others expect. Many programs and services have unstated expectations that persons with brain injury who have a history of behavioral dyscontrol are incapable of fulfilling. These expectations need not be the obvious ones (for example, following the directions of a superior), but can be subtle in nature (for example, tolerance of a certain noise level, the number of people in a room, or the time of day set for arising in the morning), to trigger behavioral outbursts. Therapists' attention to environmental manipulation in the form of reworking expectations for conformance is crucial.

"... how survivors experience the world — their phenomenology, gained from trained observation, cognitive assessment, and applied trials..."

Therapists must appreciate the world experience of persons with brain injury to successfully re-engineer their environment. It is insufficient to observe incidents of behavioral dyscontrol, only logging frequency and severity, without understanding the reasons behind it. Therapists must understand causal relationships in order to be effective when they treat high-risk behaviors.[34] Two different people with brain injury may punch a wall at an identical rate, intensity, time of day, etc. for two very different reasons. Traditional behavioral approaches that focus on behavior per se might produce identical treatment plans. However, with careful consideration of the impact of organic and neuropsychological functioning on emotions and behaviors, therapists are more likely to correctly tailor the neuropsychosocial environment to the perceptions about the world of each person with brain injury. When therapists take into account the perceptions of the world held by persons with brain injury arising from their cognitive and emotional organically derived functioning, they maximize the possibility of successful intervention. Therapists gain insight into how persons with brain injury experience the world through three primary methods.

Cognitive assessment is the foundation on which intervention is built. Thorough neuropsychological data will guide therapists in regard to how persons with brain injury attend to, perceive, reason, and retain information and events that shape their world view. Their neuropsychological information processing determines the world they experience. If persons with brain injury fail to attend to statements made to them, then those statements are not part of their world. If they reason inaccurately about an event, then it is the inaccurately drawn conclusions that are part of their world, not the theoretically correct conclusions others might appreciate. If they forget an event, there may be residual emotional shadows from it, but the event itself is no longer part of their world (though perhaps the emotional residue bears close scrutiny by therapists). A thorough neuropsychological evaluation, with interpretations designed to aid therapists in understanding the world experience of persons with brain injury, is invaluable.

Therapists with extensive experience in brain injury evaluation and care ought to be keen observers of the relationship between behavioral dyscontrol and cognitive functioning. Hence, astute trained clinical observation is the second source of knowledge about how persons with brain injury experience the world. Therapists often generate hypotheses regarding brain function and the perspective of the person with brain injury through direct observation. Important qualitative information may, in fact, only be available by attention to how the person with brain injury behaves in the real world. The value of direct observation is hard to overstate. Experienced therapists know, for example, that despite reading the medical record, nothing compares with face-to-face interview and interaction to gain insight into the motives of persons with brain injury. When forming a conceptualization of how persons with brain injury view their world, therapists must watch them interact with the world. Parenthetically, checklists, while important, should not be the sole procedure used to document information in a treatment record, because such a method does not provide insights that are captured in narrative descriptions of behavioral and psychological events.

Finally, to confirm hypotheses about how persons with brain injury conceive their world, it is crucial that therapists have the ability to change the world. Only through applied, real-world trial changes can therapists truly know whether their ideas about a person with brain injury are accurate. Thoughts about how to structure the world so that a person with brain injury will function best remain only theoretical when based solely on neuropsychological and clinical observation data. These are starting points and are the foundation on which to base a theory. However, true knowledge of the phenomenology of the person with brain injury requires hands-on adjustment of the world, with ongoing observation of the person's reaction to the changes. Therapists can confirm their understanding of a person with brain injury by awareness of how the person interprets alterations in the behavior of therapists and other people and the surrounding physical environment.

"Creation of an individualized neuropsychosocial environment..."

Therapists must create a different neuropsychosocial environment for each person with brain injury, based upon the data and the therapists' insights. For a program, this is made more difficult by the requirement to develop different neuropsychosocial environments simultaneously for different persons with brain injury, usually in the same physical space and with the same available therapists. Implementation and maintenance of different neuropsychosocial environments can be complex for residential and vocational sites. In such settings, it is helpful to have persons with brain injury who have mutually compatible neuropsychosocial treatment plans. The application of a neuropsychosocial approach in such settings will be discussed further in Chapter 7. Each person with brain injury who exhibits severe behavioral dyscontrol needs a neuropsychosocial environment that therapists tailor to the particular abilities of that person.

Creating a different neuropsychosocial environment for each person with brain injury requires that therapists behave differently with each person. Hence, therapists must intimately know the neuropsychosocial behavioral plan for each person so they can instantaneously change from one presentation, including verbal communication style, non-verbal cues, attitude, pacing, etc., to another as they turn from one person with brain injury to another. For example, saying "no" to a request from one person with brain injury might be a useful cue to help that person stop and rethink that request, but it might provoke a violent outburst when spoken to another person. In creating a neuropsychosocial environment there are no casual, off-the-record, non-therapeutic interactions.

In a program, some persons with brain injury recognize that the therapists are treating fellow persons with brain injury differently. They realize that the world their therapist provides is different for everyone. They will complain that the therapist and the treatment program are "unfair" or "unequal." Some therapists may be tempted to agree with them. Therapists may feel uncomfortable when challenged to defend inequality. However, a set approach is based on the idea of having the person with brain injury conform to program rules. Since therapists who apply a neuropsychosocial approach know that each person with brain injury requires a world tailored to the needs of the individual, they consider inequality as appropriate.

Persons with brain injury who challenge therapists about the "unfairness" of "unequal" treatment anticipate the therapists' defense of their treatment approach to be weak, since the cry of inequality places the burden on the accused therapist. Persons with brain injury are often surprised when told by experienced therapists that, "Of course you are all being treated differently. We base how we treat you on your cognitive, behavioral, and emotional abilities. Since everyone's injury is different and everyone has different goals, everyone is treated differently." Some persons with brain injury are unable to handle privileges that others can handle, but experienced therapists acknowledge the variability in abilities across persons with brain injury and avoid defensiveness in regard to the application of a different or "unequal" neuropsychosocial environment. Unequal does not imply unfair.

Therapists may also struggle with the neuropsychosocial approach when it conflicts with their preconceptions about "how people ought to behave." Society generally pushes for conformity. Therapists who have not fully studied a person with brain injury who exhibits severe behavioral dyscontrol may believe that the person should "learn" to behave in a certain way. They may even hold a moral belief in acceptable behavior and the demand to conform. Sometimes they express the view that treatment techniques should follow those that therapists use with their own unruly children. The misleading notion of basing treatment on recollections of therapists' own family dynamics and behavior was addressed by Meehl as early as 1973.[35]

Such input is usually a reflection of insufficient knowledge about brain injury. This is remediable. In many settings, education regarding brain injury and behavioral dyscontrol is inadequate. It is incumbent upon programs — whether treatment, residential, vocational, etc. — to make sure therapists avoid relying on personal experience rather than thorough training when working with persons with brain injury who exhibit behavioral dyscontrol.

Traditional approach: application/integration

The traditional model of intervention can sometimes be valuable for the care of persons with brain injury.[36] Higher level functioning persons with brain injury often present for therapy with complaints amenable to intervention with insight-oriented, contingency management, or skill-building therapies. For these individuals, the roadblocks their brain injury imposes on such treatment are few enough that a skillful therapist can help them to achieve excellent therapeutic improvement by the application of these techniques. In fact, very efficacious "outpatient" counseling uses these procedures to much advantage.

Outpatient counseling can address numerous concerns with insight-oriented, contingency management, and skill-building strategies. Emotional difficulties such as anxiety or depression often respond well to these approaches. Frequently, there are also existential issues regarding why a person was singled out for an injury: "Why me?" or where a person is going in life — "What is the purpose of living? What do I have to offer the world?" Beyond adjustment to disability issues, persons with brain injury benefit from traditional intervention for relationship rebuilding, return to work concerns, and activities of daily living challenges. Of course, even with presenting complaints such as these, the therapist must attend to cognitive variables that may interfere with treatment.

Mild behavioral problems may also respond well to the traditional treatment model. Therapists help many persons with brain injury and their families or residential care providers to address behavioral dyscontrol of a milder nature through traditional treatment methods. It is commonplace for therapists to develop behavioral plans for residential treatment sites which they structure using these procedures. These plans are often quite successful.

Even when the person with brain injury exhibits severe behavior, there is a role for the traditional model as a component of the overall neuropsychosocial approach. Some persons with brain injury may be able to benefit, at least partially, from the traditional strategies. They may be able to take advantage of these strategies for some of their problems, but not all of them, or for some degree of a problem, but not for all of it. Obviously, even in cases of severe dyscontrol, there is variable breadth and depth of a behavior and the degree to which the ability of the person with brain injury can benefit from traditional methodologies.

For the person with brain injury who primarily benefits from the neuropsychosocial approach, the utilization of traditional strategies can still be helpful for therapists in the development of a neuropsychosocial environment. Individual insight-oriented counseling, for example, may enhance a person's response to the neuropsychosocial treatment design through rapport, a sense of security, and hope. Working on skill building may promote pride and confidence. The parameters of a successful neuropsychosocial environment are frequently derived from basic work therapists do during trials of traditional strategies.

Conclusions

The neuropsychosocial approach is an innovative method for the treatment of severe behavioral dyscontrol after acquired brain injury. While it can be challenging for therapists, the rewards are tremendous. Consider a person with brain injury who is unable to exhibit behavioral control. Perhaps the person has injured other people or has assaulted a relative. The person is being kept in four-point restraints — tied down at wrists and ankles. The court system may be contemplating incarceration or state hospitalization. A now vulnerable person, who may have been an innocent victim when the brain injury occurred, suddenly faces being locked away. Now consider the alternative: there is a group of therapists who know what to do. At the conclusion of a treatment program, this person returns successfully to the community! The neuropsychosocial approach works, and its successes provide sustenance to therapists.

References

1. *Rehabilitation of Persons with Traumatic Brain Injury: NIH Consensus Statement*, National Institutes of Health, 16, 1998.
2. Fulton, D.R., Shaken baby syndrome, *Critical Care Nursing Quarterly*, 23, 43, 2000.
3. Hartman, D.E., *Neuropsychological Toxicology: Identification and Assessment of Human Neurotoxic Syndromes*, 2nd ed., Plenum Press, New York, 1995.
4. Guerrero, J.L., Thurman, D.J., and Sniezak, J.E., Emergency department visits associated with traumatic brain injury: United States, 1995–1996, *Brain Inj.*, 14, 181, 2000.
5. Thurman, D.J. et al., Traumatic brain injury in the United States: a public health perspective, *J. Head Trauma Rehab.*, 14, 602, 1999.
6. Karol, R.L., The duration of seeking help following traumatic brain injury: the persistence of symptom complaints, *The Clinical Neuropsychologist*, 3, 244, 1989.
7. Bongar, B., *The Suicidal Patient: Clinical and Legal Standards of Care*, American Psychological Association, Washington, D.C., 1991.
8. Teasdale, T.W. and Engberg, A.W., Suicidality after traumatic brain injury: a population study, *J. Neuro. Neurosurg. Psychiatry*, 71, 436, 2001.
9. *Traumatic Brain Injury Advisory Committee Annual Report 1999–2000*, Minnesota Department of Human Services, St. Paul, MN 2000.
10. Brain disorders: Minnesota's chance to keep a promise, *The Star Tribune*, Minneapolis, MN, March 18, 2001, A28.
11. Cummings, J. L., *Clinical Neuropsychiatry*, Harcourt Brace Jovanovich, New York, 1985, chap. 11.
12. Pincus, J. H., Aggression, criminality, and the frontal lobes, in *The Human Frontal Lobes: Functions and Disorders*, Miller, B.L. and Cummings, J. L., Eds., Guilford Press, New York, 1999, chap. 31.
13. Watson, D.L. and Tharp, R.G., *Self-Directed Behavior: Self-Modification for Personal Adjustment*, Brooks/Cole, Monterey, CA, 1971, chap. 3.
14. Patrick, P.D. and Hebda, D., Neurobehavioral limitations: managing aggression, *Relearning Times*, 3, 6, 1996.
15. Burke, W.H. and Lewis, F.D., Management of maladaptive social behavior of a brain injured adult, *J. Rehab.*, 9, 335, 1986.
16. Stringer, A.Y., *A Guide to Adult Neuropsychological Diagnosis*, F.A. Davis, Philadelphia, 1996, 443.
17. Turnbull, J., Perils (hidden and not so hidden) for the token economy, *J. Head Trauma Rehab.*, 3, 46, 1988.
18. Torrey, E.F., *The Mind Game: Witchdoctors and Psychiatrists*, Emerson Hall, New York, 1972.
19. *Current Procedural Terminology 2003*, American Medical Association Press, Chicago, 2002.
20. Degeneffee, C.E., Family caregiving and traumatic brain injury, *Health and Social Work*, 26, 257, 2001.
21. Frosch, S., et al., The long term effects of traumatic brain injury on the roles of caregivers, *Brain Inj.*, 11, 891, 1997.
22. Hall, K.M., et al., Family stressors in traumatic brain injury: a two-year follow-up, *Arch. Phys. Med. Rehab.*, 75, 876, 1994.

23. Leathem, J., Heath, E., and Woolley, C., Relatives' perceptions of role change, social support and stress after traumatic brain injury, *Brain Injury*, 10, 27, 1996.
24. Karol, R.L., Doerfler, L.A., Parker, J.C., and Armentrout, D.P., A therapist's manual for the cognitive-behavioral treatment of chronic pain, *JSAS Catalog of Selected Documents in Psychology*, 11, 15, 1981.
25. Hibbard, M., Psychological challenges following TBI: depression and anxiety, in Report and Recommendations from the Traumatic Brain Injury and Public Health Meeting, Atlanta, GA, 1999.
26. Langenbahn, D.M., et al., Group psychotherapy, *in Psychotherapeutic Interventions for Adults with Brain Injury or Stroke: A Clinician's Treatment Resource*, Langer, K.G., Laatsch, L., and Lewis, L., Eds., Psychosocial Press, Madison, CT, 1999, chap. 9.
27. Silver, J. M. and Yudofsky, S.C., Aggressive behavior in patients with neuropsychiatric disorders, *Neurotrauma Medical Report*, 3, 1, 1989.
28. O'Dowd, W.T., Traumatic brain injury: Toward an ecological approach to rehabilitation, presented at Traumatic Brain Injury: Tools, Trends, and Transition in the 90s, Grand Rapids, MN, May, 1992.
29. Nielsen, L., Beaver, C. and Hovdey, W., *A Systematic Approach to Maximize Recovery Via the Environment*, Idaho Elks Rehabilitation Hospital, Boise, ID, 1998.
30. Karol, R.L., Behavioral management: A neuropsychosocial approach, in Gillespie, R.A., et al., Neurobehavioral rehabilitation and community reintegration of survivors of acquired severe brain injury, presented at Brain Injury Association of Iowa Conference, Des Moines, IA, March, 1996.
31. Page, T.J., *Navigating the Curves: Behavior Changes and Brain Injury*, Brain Injury Association of America, Alexandria, VA, 1996.
32. Yody, B.B., et al., Applied behavior management and acquired brain injury: approaches and assessment, *J. Head Trauma Rehab.*, 15, 1041, 2000.
33. Matthies, B.K., Kreutzer, J. S., and West, D.D., *The Behavior Management Handbook: A Practical Approach to Patients with Neurological Disorders*, Psychological Corporation, San Antonio, TX, 1997.
34. Jacobs, H.E., *Behavior Analysis Guidelines and Brain Injury: People, Principles, and Programs*, Aspen Publishers, Gaithersburg, MD, 1993, chap. 7.
35. Meehl, P.E., Why I do not attend case conferences, in *Psychodiagnosis: Selected Papers*, P.E. Meehl, W.W. Norton, New York, chap. 13.
36. Hogan, R.T., Behavior Management for Community Reintegration, *J. Head Trauma Rehab.*, 3, 62, 1988.

chapter two

The implications of cognitive deficits for behavioral dyscontrol

Introduction

Cognitive dysfunction is the essence of brain injury. While persons with brain injury may exhibit emotional, behavioral, or physical symptoms, damage to the brain of any significant degree implies cognitive changes. In fact, the *Diagnostic and Statistical Manual of Mental Disorders–IV–TR*[1] (DSM–IV–TR), lists cognitive deficits as "the essential feature" (p. 148) of Dementia, the DSM–IV–TR's classification for significant brain injury. The DSM–IV–TR states that a diagnosis of Dementia is "characterized by multiple cognitive deficits." (p. 135), and that lesser damage, called Cognitive Disorder Not Otherwise Specified, is also "characterized by cognitive dysfunction..." (p. 136). Even delirium is "characterized by ... a change in cognition..." (p. 135). When persons with brain injury demonstrate severe behavioral dyscontrol, cognitive impairment is invariably a contributing factor. Therapists familiar with severe behavioral dyscontrol after acquired brain injury would expect cognitive impairment to be present. First, therapists are more likely to observe behavioral dyscontrol among persons with severe brain injury than among those with less significant injuries. The likelihood of behavioral dyscontrol increases with injury severity. Of course, persons with severe brain injuries are also more prone to have cognitive difficulties than those with less severe injuries. Second, the existence of cognitive deficits diminishes the brain's capacity to exert cognitive control over emotional impulses, which can lead to behavioral dyscontrol.

Numerous resources are available summarizing the array of cognitive functions (e.g., problems with attention, executive functions, memory, learning, reasoning, and language) at risk in acquired brain injury.[2,3,4] However, even when cognition is considered in relationship to behavioral dyscontrol (see Cummings [5]), attention is usually not paid to the implications of these deficits for behavioral dyscontrol in the context of treatment planning. In fact, most reviews do not attend to behavior. Rather, research considers the impact of cognitive problems on return to work or school.[6] Some research addresses the cognitive functions therapists require for persons with brain injury to drive.[7,8] Cognitive functioning is also a consideration in conservatorship and guardianship recommendations. In legal settings, lawyers and judges may weigh cognitive disturbances when making determinations about the ability of a person with brain injury to stand trial.[9]

Various authors and therapists describe how to assess and classify cognitive functioning.[10,11,12,13,14] Methods can differ from practitioner to practitioner within a discipline, and certainly can vary across disciplines. For example, "attention" can mean the ability to attend long enough to register a span of digits, or it can mean the ability to participate in a 30-minute therapy session. Both definitions are correct in their particular context, but clinically the difference between them is large. Two persons with brain injury will appear quite different if their cognitive deficit is the inability to "attend" for a few seconds or trouble persisting on task for 30 minutes.

Hence, this chapter presents cognitive problems in a manner that is useful in practice when studying cognitive determinants of behavioral dyscontrol for the applied development of clinical treatment plans. The emphasis is on the implication of cognitive dysfunction for behavioral dyscontrol, rather than a treatise on the variety of cognitive deficits, definition of terms, or classification schemes. Discussion of cognition and fundamental neuroscience or the pathophysiology underlying cognitive deficits is deferred, as other sources of such information are available to therapists.[15,16,17,18]

Cognitive functions

Orientation

Orientation refers to an awareness of self and one's surroundings. Persons with brain injury who are said to be oriented know who they are and where they are, and are aware of time; they know their name, the name of the facility they are in, the city and state, and the time, day, month, and year. They know why they are being seen by a therapist and what happened to them to bring them to the attention of the therapist or to the treatment program or facility.

Persons with brain injury who are disoriented can present a significant behavioral challenge. Disorientation can lead to irritability. When persons with brain injury are unable to accurately locate themselves in space and time, therapists may frequently reapproach them to reassess their orientation. It is frustrating for persons with brain injury to be persistently asked questions for which they do not have the answers. Of course, therapists' intentions are good, but the result may be to increase the annoyance of persons with brain injury rather than increase their orientation.

Persons with brain injury can become aggressive in response to questions they cannot answer. In addition, when persons with brain injury associate therapists with repeated questions of orientation, whether it is one particular therapist or the association is generalized to include all of their therapists, they may transfer their dislike of the experience of being disoriented to rejection of the source of the questions: the therapists. Hence, efforts to improve orientation through questioning can backfire. Noncompliance can increase. There may be a rejection of therapy. Intentional physical or verbal aggression may result, in an attempt to remove the aversive stimulus — the therapists who are perceived as annoying.

Therapists may also see an increase in confabulation in response to disorientation. Persons with brain injury attempt to make sense of their world. As the brain fills in gaps in orientation with familiar information, it constructs erroneous explanations for present experiences. Persons with brain injury can become very insistent that their world conceptualization is correct. Therapists commonly treat persons with brain injury who believe that the hospital is their place of employment and the staff are their co-workers. They believe that the hospital is a factory, office, or other job site (where they worked before their injury onset). Therapists who provide evidence to the contrary are often met with an expansion of the confabulatory scheme. Sometimes this expanded scheme incorporates the information that was supposed to help with orientation. A person with brain injury may explain that beds in the hospital are part of the lounge/rest area of a factory, or the person may explain away the orienting information: the beds are just in this section, and the rest of the factory where the person with brain injury usually works is right through a set of doors. As confabulation increases, persons with brain injury become more resistant to redirection. If they think their confabulatory scheme is correct, then it follows that they know what they are doing and therapists have no authority to restrict their activity, since the therapists were not present at the factory before.

It is more comfortable for anyone to be in familiar surroundings with a known explanation for events. Persons with brain injury are more comfortable with their confabulations than with some story told to them by strangers about brain injury and being in a hospital. From the perspectives of persons with brain injury, the problem is not that there may be some evidence that fails to fit their scheme of what is happening, but that therapists will not permit them to do what they want to do. In such instances, aggression or elopement attempts increase.

Persons with brain injury seek to assert their sense of self. They want others to perceive them as competent, functioning human beings. When therapists question something as basic as their knowledge of person, place, and time, this poses a substantial threat to their sense of competency. Thus, it should come as no surprise that persons with brain injury who lack other more sophisticated methods of rejecting an implicit message of incompetency attempt either elopement or aggression.

Attention and concentration

Attention and concentration refers to the ability to focus on the correct information long enough to allow the brain to further process it. The information may be an event, or it may be factual information of a verbal (something they read or is said to them) or nonverbal (something they see) nature. Regardless of how well the rest of the brain works, if it errs in its attention to stimuli, then information is unavailable to the brain for further processing.

Persons with brain injury who are distractible function in a world with little perceived continuity. Their world is disjointed because they miss significant bits of information, which flow past them. Moreover, disparate pieces of information are juxtaposed as persons with brain injury shift focus from what they intend to track to distracting stimuli.

Such persons with brain injury often show impairment in control of their behavior. They often demonstrate poor judgment in regard to issues of safety. Distraction leads to misjudgments, and they place themselves at risk. It is common to see persons with brain injury who are in wheelchairs and have difficulty with attention leave their wheelchair brakes unlocked when transferring in or out of the chair. They also may be unsafe in the kitchen (e.g., leaving burners on after cooking, placing sharp knives in dangerous positions, failing to clean up spills on the floor). Yet because of their cognitive impairment, they may misperceive their own abilities and insist that they are safe. Therapists' efforts to ensure safety are met with resistance.

Difficulties with attention may also lead to wandering. Persons with brain injury get lost when they attend too briefly to environmental cues that would otherwise orient them. Hence they are unable to locate their rooms, even if their names are on the door (and they can read them). Other orienting stimuli may overwhelm them rather than acting as cues, as the same stimuli might for people without brain injury. It is routine, for example, to see zones in shopping mall parking lots designated simultaneously with color, number, and animal labels (e.g., third level, green elephant) to maximize cues. This also helps persons with brain injury, but the number of cues may lead them to reach their saturation point sooner than it would for people without brain injury.

Distractibility can increase demanding behavior. If persons with brain injury make requests to their therapists and then fail to attend to the answer, the persons with brain injury become annoyed. Their annoyance reflects that their brain never had the chance to process the answer because they were distracted. Highly inattentive persons with brain injury are frequently intrusive since they ask questions, pay little attention to the answers, and then re-approach to inquire again. As they repeat this cycle, irritability rises and they eventually lash out in frustration.

Therapists can observe a rise in social inappropriateness due to poor concentration. Persons with brain injury miss contextual social cues for appropriate behavior. Social interaction requires attention to a highly complicated and continually shifting set of variables, and these factors are different in each situation. Even when superficial appearances make situations seem like a repeat of past interactions, one variable being different can alter the whole event. Attention to this kaleidoscope of information is very hard. After an event of dyscontrol, persons with brain injury may report not having noticed a social signal that the therapist is now highlighting for them.

Executive functions

Executive functions subsume diverse cognitive tasks. Impairment of these functions leads to problems in tracking, sequencing, self-monitoring, responding to feedback, and problem solving. There can be difficulties with initiation, perseveration, and impulsivity.

The inability to track and sequence can be exasperating for persons with brain injury. They may focus on a discussion or activity but be incapable of sustaining it. Hence, their performance declines over the course of an interaction. They may make errors by doing something out of order or losing track of what they were doing. Their ineffectualness tests their resolve, and their disappointment in themselves can be the occasion for anger directed at themselves or other people. When they turn the anger on themselves, therapists will see depression, guilt, and self-destructive behavior. When they display their anger toward other people, they place others at risk for physical harm. Moreover, the unreliability of persons with brain injury may make other people angry. When persons with brain injury detect the anger of other people, it can provoke an emotional response in turn by the persons with brain injury.

In addition, due to inadequate self-monitoring, persons with brain injury may be unaware of their errors. They may believe that their own conduct is fine, when it really falls short. Those around them, of course, base their judgments about the person with brain injury on actual performance, which may not match with the perceptions of the person with brain injury who omits self-monitoring. Because other people base decisions regarding the privileges and responsibilities they allow a person with brain injury to have on their own judgments, the mismatch between the view of the person with brain injury and the conceptualization of others brings about resentment in the person with brain injury. This resentment fuels behavioral outbursts, since the person with brain injury cannot understand why others judge their performance as insufficient. Failure to self-monitor leaves the person with brain injury with the perception that the world is unfair.

Inadequate self-monitoring leads to poor problem solving. Problem solving requires people to become aware that a problem exists through tracking over time. Next, they must attend to details to recognize the nature of the problem. Then they must generate alternative solutions and weigh the likelihood for success against possible side effects of each solution. After implementation of a solution, problem solving requires re-evaluation to determine the outcome of solution implementation and what adjustments must be made.[19] This very complex procedure befuddles persons with brain injury if they are incapable of good executive functioning. Therefore, they are less able to cope with people and events. Depression may increase, as may aggravation with a world they cannot handle.

Many persons with brain injury who have difficulties with behavioral control respond poorly when given feedback. In part, this is because they perceive their own skills and their skill implementation to be fine. Also, they may withhold recognition of the right to comment on their performance from the people who actually do have a responsibility to guide them. Nobody likes being told about their shortcomings from someone who they feel has little authority to comment on their actions. In an effort to be left alone by people providing feedback, persons with brain injury may physically strike out and attack them.

Some persons with brain injury may acknowledge the appropriateness of feedback and guidance but persist in making mistakes. Perseveration causes repetition of wrong responses. When other people become upset by the discrepancies between what persons with brain injury say and what they do, persons with brain injury respond with a loss of behavioral control. Moreover, perseveration can cause not just a relapse to mistaken responses in situations but also to an inability to relinquish an erroneous idea or belief.

Continual assertion of an incorrect idea is also wearing on other people. Since persons with brain injury commonly wish to act on their ideas, as does everyone, therapists may need to intervene to protect persons with brain injury from themselves. Again, this can be the source for significant behavioral disputes.

Impulsivity occurs when the brain either overly activates responses or undercontrols activity. Impulsivity normally demands the attention of therapists because of the risk of harm to the person with brain injury or to someone else. An array of behavioral difficulties arises from impulsivity, including poor safety decision-making (e.g., unassisted, risky wheelchair transfers), social and sexual inappropriateness (e.g., badly chosen comments, touching), elopement, or suicide. On the other hand, persons with brain injury can also demonstrate trouble with initiation. They fail to start activities. They are passive. While passivity generally commands less attention from therapists than impulsivity, it nevertheless can be the origin of behavioral problems.

Noncompliance can have its roots in passivity. Persons with brain injury may come up short in their fulfillment of obligations. For example, they may socially withdraw, becoming isolated and depressed. They can become a drain on the energy level of other people who strive to motivate them. This eventually frustrates other people, causing them to be angry with the person with brain injury, or it can lead other people to have progressively fewer interactions with the person with brain injury.

Even the passive person with a brain injury may show irritation at being ignored or left out of activities. As a result, other people may become angry or withdraw, and the person with brain injury becomes isolated, depressed, and irritable. This combination is a tinderbox for an eventual behavioral explosion in a seemingly docile person with brain injury. Therapists with experience in behavioral dyscontrol easily recognize stories of passive persons with brain injury who suddenly explode in anger. The uninformed observer of such an explosion can be quite surprised at the vehemence with which such an outburst can occur.

Memory and learning

The exemplar of cognitive dysfunction after acquired brain injury, in addition to executive function limitations, is disruption of memory and learning. Persons with brain injury of any substantial degree, by definition, suffer alteration in memory functioning.[1] Memory and learning are complex, and their disruption triggers behavioral dyscontrol.

When persons with brain injury have memory problems, they tend to live in "the here and now." They lose continuity over time as they struggle to remember what has been said or what has occurred. When they forget plans for the future and are unable to recall what is going to happen next, it becomes natural to focus on current conversations and ongoing events. However, this can cause considerable problems. Uninjured people make decisions based upon past experience in anticipation of future considerations. If persons with brain injury only have available for cognitive processing "here and now" variables, the choices of other people will seem inconsistent, and perhaps worse, capricious. Other people have more information on which to choose a course of action, which may impact upon persons with a brain injury.

Persons with brain injury lose the historical context of events or statements. It is easy to be upset when there is little appreciation of how something came to pass. Without background information available through memory storage and access, it is easy to be distressed and lose control. If each event or interaction must stand alone, then it is impossible for persons with brain injury to have their perspectives evolve over time. Hence, when they encounter a restriction imposed by therapists, the restriction makes no sense. They forget the behavior that led to the limitation. The actions the therapists take appear arbitrary and unreasonable. For example, if therapists restrict a person with brain injury from going on an outing because of behavioral difficulties during the last outing, and the person with brain injury cannot recall the behavioral dyscontrol, then the prohibition from participating in the new outing appears unjustified. Similarly, in the real world, persons with brain injury who forget significant information are unable to appreciate why other people act in regard to them as they do. Past conversations and actions are lost to memory deficit.

Persons with brain injury show increased dyscontrol when others treat them in a manner that presents as unfair. This unfairness may, in fact, only be in the eye of the person with brain injury, since to everyone else the treatment is appropriate, given variables forgotten by the person with brain injury. Persons with brain injury are frequently unable to appreciate the impact of their forgotten behavior on other people. They can lose diverse types of information, including conversations, agreements, and plans. People who attempt to hold persons with brain injury to agreements may absorb the brunt of behavioral dyscontrol. When persons with brain injury react to other people's insistence on agreements which they fail to remember, behavioral dyscontrol can easily escalate.

A simple example demonstrates this point. A family tells a person with a brain injury that after the person's appointment is over, the person should "call us and we will pick you up." After the appointment, the person with brain injury sits in the lobby awaiting the family member's arrival. Having forgotten two words, "call us," the person with a brain injury never calls. After an hour or so, the family comes looking for the loved one. A verbal fight follows in the lobby. The person with brain injury spent the hour getting progressively angrier since no one came. The family, in the meantime, became worried and anxious. An explosion ensues as the angry person with brain injury encounters an anxious, stressed family. The person with brain injury accuses the family of not caring. The anger is about the broken promise of "we will pick you up." This accusation stresses the family members who recall also saying, "call us," which the person with the brain injury forgot. This acrimony is a function of the memory deficit. Two small words, remembered or forgotten, have led to aggression, mistrust, and accusations.

Memory and learning deficits also hinder treatment. Chapter 1 discussed the broad implications of memory and learning deficits for insight-oriented, skill-building, and contingency management therapies. However, even in a neuropsychosocial approach, the retention of environmental information can facilitate behavioral improvement. For example, consider a young male who inappropriately touches women in a sexual manner when the women visit his residence to see another person with brain injury. Initial treatment efforts might focus on insight regarding women and their responses to such sexualized behavior. Additional therapy might entail social skills training of alternative behaviors. If insufficient progress occurs and the behavior persists, a neuropsychosocial approach could entail decreased access to others' visitors. In this fashion, the behavior will not occur since the person with brain injury who demonstrates inappropriate sexual behavior is no longer allowed contact with the women he targets. However, such a neuropsychosocial change is more likely to be accepted if the person with brain injury remembers why the therapists instituted access restrictions. The neuropsychosocial change will stop the behavior whether or not the person with brain injury remembers why therapists imposed it, but better memory functioning will ease implementation.

Verbal reasoning

The ability to think using language permits the processing of complex information. When this ability is damaged after acquired brain injury, persons with brain injury lose the capacity to fully appreciate and process information. This loss influences both intake and output of information. Comprehension declines, as does the generation of complex ideas. Poor verbal reasoning exacerbates behavioral dyscontrol. Requests to persons with brain injury who have lowered verbal reasoning are misunderstood. Instructions make less sense. Explanations are of less value. Therapists or others (family members, for example) must simplify information, but some topics are difficult to make elementary. If a subject is impossible to sufficiently simplify, then persons with brain injury operate with only partial data as they make decisions.

Behavioral dyscontrol easily stems from poor verbal reasoning. Either facts and opinions are misunderstood or a topic is too complex to absorb. Both of these problems leave persons with brain injury with less knowledge than others have on which to base their actions. When persons with brain injury lack the ability to verbally reason, their ideas may lack sophistication and fall short of necessary thoroughness or subtlety. Hence, when persons with brain injury assert their desires, other people may reject their suggestions because a better course of action seems advisable with fuller reasoning. Left with desires but inadequate skill at verbal explanation to win over other people to their ideas and achieve implementation, persons with brain injury may lash out. Anger, mistrust, and dyscontrol result when the ideas of persons with brain injury are rejected.

Language functioning

Many persons with brain injury have difficulty with language functioning. They may have problems with oral and written expression and reception of information. Such problems can include fundamental language processing as well as motor disturbances. Persons with brain injury can find receptive and expressive communication challenges to be some of the most frustrating changes they face because so much of human interaction is based on oral and written exchanges. When persons with brain injury have limits on their communication, they can have extraordinary deficiencies in their relationships with other people. They can feel isolated and alone. They are left out of conversations. They can become depressed. They may strike out in frustration or for attention.

People are often in a hurry during conversation, and persons with brain injury who have language hurdles frequently require extra time to formulate conversation. Plus, they must be able to marshal their concentration to track a conversation. For example, spelling boards or devices that speak after persons with brain injury type in words necessitate a great amount of attention on the part of persons with brain injury to accomplish even simple communication. When other people fail to provide sufficient effort or time to help overcome communication problems, persons with brain injury experience a great deal of frustration. This is particularly true when persons with brain injury otherwise have ample cognitive function, for example, memory and verbal reasoning capacities, to comprehend communication and to formulate a good response.

Therapists should anticipate anger on the part of persons with brain injury when other people inadequately assist in communication. Grabbing people to try to obtain their attention and to detain them to finish conversation is common. When frustrated, persons with brain injury may throw or hit their assistive communication device, out of anger. They may demonstrate noncompliance through refusal to further use an assistive device.

Nonverbal reasoning/perceptual skills

For most uninjured people, it is hard to conceptualize thought without words. Nevertheless, people process a large amount of information without language. This can be noticeably evident after brain injury. If persons with brain injury cannot understand nonverbal information, they are at a significant disadvantage when they attempt to relate to other people. Nonverbal cues and communication are essential to fully understand interactions and events. People often grasp context and thereby gain insight about meaning though nonverbal reasoning. Nonverbal reasoning and perceptual skills facilitate appreciation of context. Statements people make may have different meanings in different situations, and situational variables are commonly nonverbal in nature. Uninjured people may use nonverbal signals to supplement their words, and persons with brain injury may miss these signals. Uninjured people may also use nonverbal signs when persons with brain injury are speaking, to show a response to what they have heard. Persons with brain injury tend to miss cues about how the other person feels about what is being said.

Persons with brain injury can have difficulty in their own use of nonverbal information as well. They may send incongruent nonverbal cues when they speak, confusing their listeners. When they listen to others, they may show nonverbal cues about their thoughts, which are erroneous. Finally, persons with brain injury may communicate well, but provide their message in the wrong setting, to the wrong people, at the wrong time.

Both receptive and expressive interactions require good nonverbal skills for maximum effectiveness: persons with brain injury may have difficulty communicating because of nonverbal reasoning/perceptual problems. Such failures lead to behavioral dyscontrol. Verbal processing problems are usually easily recognizable, but nonverbal difficulties may be hidden. Meaning is lost and misunderstanding increases, resulting in behavioral dyscontrol.

Behavioral dyscontrol due to nonverbal processing problems can be particularly troublesome because of the less obvious nature of the nonverbal processing problem. The behavioral difficulties stemming from nonverbal processing problems are more likely to appear to uninformed observers as having little foundation, and thus the rapidity or severity of the behavior startles the recipient of aggression. Chart notes often have entries describing unprovoked dyscontrol. The dyscontrol may be judged to be more severe than it would otherwise be rated because of the observer's surprise at its occurrence. Normally, if aggression is anticipated, action can be taken to dispel the causes or mitigate its impact. When people experience dyscontrol directed at them for which they are unprepared, they determine it to have been more severe than if they had anticipated it.

Mechanical skills/motor skills

The brain controls the physical body. It determines the ability to move through space, organize physical responses, and manipulate objects. Uninjured people take their physical prowess for granted. Loss of control over one's body can be devastating.

Physical disability can impair mobility. Some persons with brain injury require a wheelchair or walker. Some can adequately ambulate, but may do so slowly. In either case, limitations in mobility impair one's ability to easily participate in activities. Thus, even when persons with brain injury make the effort to participate in activities, these physical challenges can effect spontaneity. As a result, social isolation may develop as a function of mobility problems. Some persons with brain injury demonstrate increasing helplessness and dependency beyond that which their mobility difficulty imposes. Despair can increase. The disturbance in emotional status due to social isolation from mobility hurdles can trigger behavioral dyscontrol.

Motor skill deficits can cause awkwardness when trying to accomplish a chore. The tasks that these deficits can affect range from control of a pen for writing to activities of daily living (for example, eating, dressing, or toileting) to social activities (for example, swimming, bowling, or dancing). Persons with brain injury may finish the activity, but in a disorganized manner. They may be unable to complete a task at all. The privilege of driving is at risk when persons with brain injury have impairment in motor control. All of these limitations impact the self-image of persons with brain injury and can be a continual source of frustration. The likelihood for behavioral outbursts increases when persons with brain injury are constantly frustrated.

The importance of cognitive assessment for treatment implementation

It is essential that therapists have access to good cognitive evaluation data when dealing with behavioral dysfunction after acquired brain injury. Appropriate cognitive information about persons with brain injury is important because cognitive deficits account for much of the probability that behavioral dyscontrol will occur. Moreover, cognitive functioning influences the nature of the dyscontrol therapists may observe. Treatment strategies must be based on the cognitive capabilities of the person with brain injury in order to devise successful interventions. This is true for traditional treatment methodologies as well.[20]

Therapists in treatment programs that address behavioral dyscontrol often receive referrals to treat persons with brain injury who have never received appropriate cognitive assessment. Sometimes there is a history of years of failed treatment with no adequate determination of the person's cognitive functioning. These referrals are often accompanied by extensive and carefully detailed behavioral plans which have failed. Treatment failure is often due to previous therapists' poor conceptualization of the nature of cognitive disturbances that underlie behavioral dyscontrol. Too much time is spent writing complex treatment plans which lack foundation in the cognitive abilities of the person with brain injury. More time should be devoted to cognitive evaluation, and therapists who write treatment plans should understand the implications of the individual's cognitive strengths and weaknesses before writing the plan.

Of course, excellent therapists can make judgments about individual cases using astute clinical understanding of behavioral observations to work backwards to an appreciation of fundamental underlying cognitive functioning. Nevertheless, good cognitive evaluation should be the standard procedure when possible. It is too easy for less knowledgeable or less observant therapists to insufficiently discern cognitive functioning.

The types of cognitive evaluations that therapists obtain are important. Many evaluations provide comprehensive data with little consideration given to treatment planning for behavioral dyscontrol. It is paramount that the assessor conceptualize the data for the therapists in a manner that is clinically useful. Cognitive evaluators must tailor their assessments to be applicable to treatment design for behavioral dyscontrol.

For many rehabilitation disciplines, orienting assessments and reports for the purpose of behavioral dyscontrol treatment planning is difficult. Neuropsychologists who have not directly provided therapy can have a poor understanding of the type of cognitive information and interpretation that therapists require. An evaluation typical of a neuropsychological diagnostic testing laboratory service in a large research hospital focused primarily on diagnosis and localization is likely to be inadequate for behavioral treatment planning. The report and its interpretation may lack clinical treatment relevance. Similarly, other disciplines (e.g., occupational therapy, speech/language pathology) can also have trouble adjusting their orientation to assess persons with brain injury with behavioral dyscontrol. The data necessary for constructing a treatment plan for activities of daily living or communication may be different than the cognitive data occupational therapists or speech language pathologists need to determine how not to get hit by persons with brain injury.

Building a treatment plan for behavioral dyscontrol mandates that therapists have cognitive data which either they or another evaluator conceptualize to understand the cognitive foundation of behavioral dyscontrol. Fortunately, there are evaluators and therapists across disciplines who can do this, but it requires specially trained professionals experienced with behavioral dyscontrol. Novice therapists may make theoretical statements about cognitive difficulties and their implications for behavioral problems without first-hand experience dealing with truly dangerous dyscontrol. Therapists must have the opportunity to learn whether following their conceptualizations results in a decline in behavioral dyscontrol. Feedback is crucial so that evaluators can adjust how they translate raw data into treatment recommendations.

These specially trained professionals must decide that they *want* to work with behavioral dyscontrol. Since the interpretation of cognitive data when working with behavioral dyscontrol is different from that found in traditional settings and the treatment tasks are different from what is typically taught to most disciplines, therapists need to be comfortable with a new way to conceive their role. Professionals across disciplines who provide cognitive interpretations, and therapy based upon them, should prepare themselves for occasional askance comments or lack of emotional support from colleagues who lack appreciation of the nature of this non-traditional application of professional cognitive data interpretation.

The following example shows how data needs to be interpreted in a behavioral treatment program setting. Suppose that cognitive testing reveals that a person with brain injury has difficulty in mental control, particularly when a task requires simultaneous attention to multiple items. The data also shows slow processing speed. The person's language functioning is adequate for conversation, but there is mild impairment in verbal reasoning. Nonverbal reasoning is impaired. Reports indicate that the person with brain injury has a history of behavioral dysfunction when approached by someone asking a question, but this is inconsistent. To address this problem, an interpretation of cognitive data that focuses on confirmation of the brain injury diagnosis or localization of damage to correlate with radiographic studies will be insufficient for behavioral treatment planning. A skilled therapist, however, will be able to integrate behavioral observations with cognitive data.

In this case example a careful, thorough behavioral observation is very informative. Initially, therapists note that the outbursts seem more common when other people are around. Further study determines that they occur when one of these people is having a conversation with the person with brain injury. Eventually, therapists find that the dyscontrol occurs when additional people approach to join the conversation.

Interpretation of cognitive test results with a perspective on behavioral dyscontrol helps explain the person's behavioral dyscontrol. The person with brain injury has difficulty tracking multiple sources of information. Hence, when additional speakers join a conversation, information overload occurs. Slow processing speed compounds the problem. One speaker may slow down to match the capability of the person with brain injury, but multiple speakers in a group begin matching each other's conversation rate, leaving the person with brain injury behind. Since the person with brain injury has sufficient language and verbal reasoning skill to participate in one-on-one conversation, as opposed to withdrawal from conversation because of consistent inadequacies in communication, the person with brain injury knows that the ability to converse is present. The person in our example has high expectations and is frustrated when others intrude. Because of poor nonverbal processing, the person with brain injury cannot tell when an approaching individual intends to interrupt to ask a brief question or to join the discussion. The person with brain injury, tired of long interruptions or others joining an ongoing conversation, reacts with irritability to even a brief interruption. Anger and dyscontrol, founded in cognitive deficits, escalates.

Behavioral observations alone will not lead to a good treatment plan. By themselves, behavioral observations in the above case might have led people to have less conversation with the person with brain injury. However, combined with cognitive test data a number of treatment options become apparent. People wishing to speak with the person with brain injury could stand aside and wait for the current conversation to end. Perhaps they could even approach the people in the current conversation, including the person with brain injury, and not talk until a break in the discussion occurred. At that point, the person talking would need to know to be quiet or step back to allow the person with brain injury to attend to the new speaker. In addition, new speakers could use a predetermined signal agreed to by the person with brain injury when they need to approach to ask a question (e.g., a note card that says, "Brief Question Only" or a key word or phrase to use). Finally, perhaps initial conversations with this person with brain injury could be initiated when and where there will be little chance of interruption. Conversations could take place in a private room rather than in common areas. A speaker could inquire of others nearby about whether they need to talk with the person with brain injury prior to the speaker starting a new conversation.

The preceding example is overly simplistic, but illustrates the point that behavioral observations need to be integrated with cognitive data. The methodologies are endless once behavioral and cognitive data come together. Of course, after implementation of any plan, ongoing adjustment to the initial conceptualizations and plans is necessary as successes and setbacks lead to refinement.

Conclusions

Behavioral dyscontrol typically has cognitive underpinnings. Treatment planning for behavioral dyscontrol after brain injury requires therapists to contemplate how cognitive deficits lead to behavioral dyscontrol. All types of cognitive deficits can trigger behavioral problems. The challenge therapists have is to appreciate the implications of cognitive dysfunction and to match cognitive data with behavioral observations. Only by synthesizing cognitive and behavioral information can therapists devise good treatment plans.

References

1. *Diagnostic and Statistical Manual of Mental Disorders*, 4th ed., Text Revision, American Psychiatric Association, Washington, D.C., 2000.
2. Miller, B.L. and Cummings, J. L., Eds., *The Human Frontal Lobes: Functions and Disorders*, Guilford Press, New York, 1999.
3. Williamson, D.J.G., Scott, J. G., and Adams, R.L., Traumatic brain injury, in *Neuropsychology for Clinical Practice: Etiology, Assessment, and Treatment of Common Neurological Disorders*, Adams, R.L., et al., Eds., American Psychological Association, Washington, D.C., 1996.
4. Zakzanis, K.K., Leach, L., and Kaplan, E., *Neuropsychological Differential Diagnosis*, Swets & Zeitlinger, Exton, PA, 1999.
5. Cummings, J. L., *Clinical Neuropsychiatry*, Harcourt Brace Jovanovich, New York, 1985, Chap.6.
6 Ip, R.Y., Dornan, J., and Schentag, C., Traumatic brain injury: factors predicting return to work or school, *Brain Injury*, 9, 517, 1995.
7. Coleman, R.D. et al., Predictors of driving outcome after traumatic brain injury, *Arch. Phys. Med Rehab.*, 83, 1415, 2002.
8. Schultheis, M.T. and Rizzo, A.A., New directions in neuropsychology: virtual reality technology, *American Psychological Association Division of Clinical Neuropsychology Newsletter*, 40, 20, 3, 2002.
9. Blau, T.H., *The Psychologist as Expert Witness*, John Wiley & Sons, New York, 1984, Chapter 6.
10. Crawford, J. R., Parker, D.M. and McKinlay, W.W., Eds., *A Handbook of Neuropsychological Assessment*, Lawrence Erlbaum Associates, Hove, UK, 1992.
11. Lezak, M.D., *Neuropsychological Assessment*, 3rd ed., Oxford University Press, New York, 1995.
12. Mitrushina, M.N., Boone, K.B., and D'Elia, L.F., *Handbook of Normative Data for Neuropsychological Assessment*, Oxford University Press, New York, 1999.
13. Reeves, D. and Wedding, D., *The Clinical Assessment of Memory: A Practical Guide*, Springer Publishing Company, New York, 1994.
14. Spreen, O. and Strauss, E., *A Compendium of Neuropsychological Tests*, 2nd ed., Oxford University Press, New York, 1998.
15. Bannister, R., *Brain's Clinical Neurology*, 5th ed., Oxford University Press, New York, 1978.
16. Beatty, J., *The Human Brain: Essentials of Behavioral Neuroscience*, Sage Publications, Thousand Oaks, CA, 2001.
17. Lundy-Ekman, L., *Neuroscience: Fundamentals for Rehabilitation*, 2nd ed., W.B. Saunders, New York, 2002.
18. Luria, A.R., *Higher Cortical Functions in Man*, 2nd ed., Basic Books, New York, 1980.
19. D'Zurilla, T.J. and Goldfried, M.R., Problem solving and behavior modification. *J. Abnormal Psychol.*, 78, 107, 1971.
20. O'Neill, H., *Managing Anger*, Whurr Publishers, London, UK, 1999.

chapter three

The contribution of adjustment issues to behavioral dyscontrol

Introduction

Therapists must understand both the nature of the adjustment issues persons with brain injury face and the implications for behavioral dyscontrol when those issues remain unresolved. Therapists who attend only to cognitive and physical deficits after brain injury and downplay emotional concerns are unlikely to ameliorate behavioral dyscontrol. However, the zeitgeist of our health care system affects therapists' attention to issues of adjustment.

Two competing trends in health care tug on the direction of care for persons with brain injury. Therapists are increasingly acknowledging the importance of emotional issues and the perspectives on life of persons with brain injury post onset. For example, the Commission on Accreditation of Rehabilitation Facilities (CARF) has set standards that utilize a person-centered approach and use language directed at "the person served."[1] These standards recognize that how persons with brain injury perceive events and feel about them, including their own rehabilitation, must be paramount in treatment. However, reimbursement sources seek to control costs by paying for the minimum care necessary for survival outside of a treatment facility. Unfortunately, there is an extensive gap between the global needs of the person served and the minimal requirements necessary to survive. In this gulf lie issues of emotional adjustment. In the case of behavioral dyscontrol after brain injury, there is no choice but to address emotional issues since without treatment of adjustment concerns, behavioral outbursts result. In that regard, survival does require treatment of emotional problems, as society is intolerant of the behavior that will result when treatment of emotional status is deferred.

Etiology of adjustment issues

Persons with brain injury face a myriad of adjustment concerns. Therapists can gain an appreciation for this not just by noting the professional literature, but by reading books written by persons with brain injury or their family members.[2,3,4,5] Compared to people experiencing other disabilities, persons with brain injury must cope with the fallout from loss of function of the brain. It is the brain that is damaged: the overall control center for everything a person does. Damage to the brain spares little.

There are numerous ways in which people present a sense of accomplishment to the world and in doing so help establish their own sense of self-worth. For example, some people cope with life through financial prowess. They take pride in their monetary success. They spend time working and enjoy the financial benefits of their efforts. They often cope with challenges in life by using their wealth to solve problems. Unfortunately, after brain injury financial status changes. Many persons with brain injury are unable to return to work, even after rehabilitation. Other persons return to work at a much lower rate of pay. Sometimes, difficulty in returning to work is a reflection of an inadequate supply of job training, placement, and coaching services from therapists with expertise in brain injury. Using a general job service or vocational agency to help persons with brain injury get a job is likely to fail, because the staff at such generic providers is usually unaware of the implications of cognitive difficulties after acquired brain injury.

The overall household income of persons with brain injury may drop from circumstances other than that person's lost wages. Spouses may see a decline in their own earnings if they were earning a separate income prior to the onset of the brain injury. Early in treatment, spouses frequently take time off of work to be at the hospital and, later, the rehabilitation center. When persons with brain injury return home the support services spouses must provide often prevent them from either a partial or full-time return to work. Hence, just when spousal income may be most necessary, it decreases or disappears.

Other financial resources may prove to be less than expected. Government disability payments are usually lower than persons with brain injury anticipate. Legal settlements may be too low for potential lifelong needs. Too few people have disability policies, and even if they do have them, they may find that they are insufficient.[6,7] Many policies have restricted definitions of disability or definitions of return to work that are too broad. Thus, policies may refuse to pay for the loss of a high-paying job if one qualifies for menial work. Many policies offer short-term coverage or offer long-term coverage for only a limited number of years, rather than providing payment to retirement age.

Some people handle the world through their physical skills. They use their physical prowess to present an image to the world. Their job choice may reflect their physical strength, speed, and dexterity. At home, perhaps they take pride in "handy-man" skills. Recreational time might be spent in a home shop, fixing their cars and homes, or at a hobby building things from crafts to furniture.

The increase in athletic participation for preventative health reasons in the last few decades has resulted in more people using athletic skills to define themselves. Social and recreational time is devoted to athletic pursuits. From the "weekend warrior" to the compulsive jogger or bicyclist to the exercisers who fill corporate gyms at lunchtime, many people develop a physical and psychological self-image intertwined with their athletic activities.

Physical skills can diminish when people experience brain injury. Visuopractic and visuospatial deficits are common results of brain injury. Impulsivity, poor planning, and tracking deficits contribute to inferior execution of physical activities. Alterations in sensory functioning, such as visual changes, are frequent symptoms of brain injury. Spasticity and paralysis are also seen after brain injury. Some people need wheelchairs. Some have balance and coordination problems or slower motor speed. Equipment (e.g., sports gear, camping equipment) is often insufficiently engineered for people with disabilities. All of these problems may prevent persons with brain injury from using physical competency and athletics to build self-worth.

Some people use their fortunate good looks and sexual prowess to define themselves. One need not be a runway model to base one's life on one's physical appearance. From simple pride in how one dresses to being "hot" into the dating scene, appearance is a tool people use to define themselves. This may be considerably more difficult after brain injury. Scars from injury onset or surgery can be difficult to mask. Physical disability can impair one's outward appearance. Money concerns can restrict access to fashion and nightlife. Mobility challenges such as dependency on wheelchairs or canes and restrictions on driving can affect participation in social activities and the maintenance of a positive self-image.

Finally, many people handle life by being smart. They obtain jobs predicated on education. They rise through business by solving problems. Intellectual pursuits define their social lives. Obviously, brain injury with its cognitive impairments can affect intelligence. Attention, reasoning, language, and memory functioning are at risk after brain injury. Hence, many of the abilities people use to achieve a sense of self-efficacy can be lost after brain injury.

In contrast to brain injury, other disabilities do not necessarily have an impact on so many aspects of how people establish their self-worth. For example, after spinal cord injury, unless there is an undiagnosed concomitant brain injury, intelligence is unaffected. Brain injury affects so many abilities that it is hardly surprising that persons with brain injury face tremendous issues of adjustment.

Cognition and adjustment

There is an obvious link between cognitive dysfunction and issues of adjustment. In addition to having to adjust *to* cognitive deficits, persons with brain injury must adjust *with* cognitive deficits: they must cope with the life changes that brain injury imposes upon them with a brain that processes information poorly. Inattention, lowered comprehension, and inadequate memory cause persons with brain injury to have a difficult time adjusting to life and its challenges.

Persons with brain injury have limited coping resources because they mishandle information. They may forget to use available assistance, or they may lose the information that resources have provided. They may misunderstand helpful communication or they may try to apply therapeutic information in a distorted fashion. Successful coping requires problem solving, and persons with brain injury find it difficult to problem-solve with forgotten or distorted information. They find it challenging to apply even correctly learned and remembered insights and skills when they perceive situations inaccurately and make erroneous attributions. Hence, cognitive deficits make coping efforts ineffective. Persons with brain injury spiral downward into increasing frustration as their attempts to cope and adjust are thwarted by cognitive difficulties.

In the context of injury to the body's most vital organ, persons with brain injury must struggle to find meaning, hope, and purpose. These existential variables are difficult to wrestle with when the body part that contemplates existential issues is damaged. Thinking and reflecting is hard when the thinking and reflecting organ works incorrectly.

Adjustment issues

Depression

The challenges that persons with brain injury confront every day can be overwhelming. As noted previously, the losses can easily lead to a diminished sense of self-esteem and self-worth. Persons with brain injury who experience an increase in self-deprecation are at risk for depression.

Persons with brain injury experience the full range of depressive symptoms seen in other populations. As discussed, they have much to be depressed about and may lack sufficient resources to cope. It is beyond the scope of this chapter to delineate depressive symptomology (for example, see Beck, et al.[8]), but it is essential to realize that depression can be the foundation for behavioral dyscontrol.

Persons with brain injury who are depressed can be irritable. They are frustrated and often angry. Attempts by therapists to engage them are met with resistance. In part, the resistance is a reflection of their belief that life is terrible with their injury and that, since the therapist cannot change the injury, life will continue to be awful. So, they despair of any positive change occurring through treatment. Their desire to be left alone represents a belief that they are, at least temporarily, more comfortable emotionally in their anguish than they will be if they let a therapist stir things up. Since they have been unable to solve life's challenges due to their brain injury and they may not appreciate the shortcomings in their efforts because their brain did not signal them appropriately when they made mistakes in problem solving, they believe that the therapists' attempts to help them will be no better than their own trials. In such circumstances, therapy efforts are likely to be just one more annoyance they must confront after brain injury.

Behavioral dyscontrol can reflect depression. Depression can easily cause resistance and noncompliance. If therapists target these behaviors without paying sufficient attention to underlying depression they can actually cause them to worsen, turning resistance and noncompliance to actual aggression.

Anxiety/fear

Persons with brain injury who exhibit behavioral dyscontrol are often anxious and afraid. The world is complex and they have difficulty keeping up. Fearfulness stems from not understanding what is happening, or forgetting what has already occurred. These people may not recall what they have been told is going to happen next, and they cannot figure it out on their own. Fear and anxiety arise from their uncertainty about other people and the world. In addition, some persons with brain injury may experience post-traumatic stress disorder.[9]

Fearful and anxious persons with brain injury are often uncooperative. They may fail to agree with helpful plans. They may misperceive the intent of others. When therapists or other people attempt to get physically or emotionally close to persons with brain injury, they lash out verbally or physically because they are afraid. For example, they may fear physical harm during activity of daily living care, or they may experience anxiety when asked to be emotionally trusting.

To cope with anxiety and fear, persons with brain injury may physically strike out to drive people away who make them feel uncomfortable. If physical aggression does not remove those people who are irritants, or if the persons with brain injury are not inclined toward exhibition of physical aggression to achieve their goals, they may attempt to elope. In either instance, they are seeking to reduce anxiety and discomfort by changing their environment.

Persons with brain injury who are afraid also tend to decrease their anxiety by seeking control. One way to be in control is to be isolative. When persons with brain injury withdraw, they create a universe where they are less fearful. Withdrawal is often both physical and social. By having less contact with other people and staying in environments that are familiar and over which they have mastery, they are able to keep anxiety in check.

In addition, persons with brain injury may seek to have control over material resources. In an effort to avoid depending upon others, they may gather things that help them feel more secure. If they perceive the world as unreliable and scary to deal with, hoarding behavior may occur. Frequently hoarded items include paper, writing implements, magazines, catalogs, food, and even drinking straws.

Suicidality

Persons with brain injury are at greater risk for suicide than other people because of the increased likelihood of the presence of suicide risk factors. Suicide risk correlates with, among other factors, depression, poor problem solving, and hopelessness.[10] These factors are readily observable in persons with brain injury.

Depression, as noted, is common among persons with brain injury. They may believe that because their injury has resulted in a chronic, incurable condition, their life situation is similarly unfixable. (In part, of course, they believe life can be no better because they are poor problem solvers due cognitive impairment.) Hence, they are at risk for suicide.

Many persons with brain injury are impulsive due to damage to areas of the brain responsible for executive functions. Impulsivity increases the risk for suicide because impulsive people act precipitously. Sometimes they simply wish to signal a cry for help, but because of their impulsivity actually choose a method that is more lethal than they really intend and kill themselves by mistake.

Chemical use is an additional consideration in suicide risk. It can distort judgment, impairing problem solving, and can increase depression.[11] Chemical use can enhance disinhibition, raising impulsivity. Chemical abuse that impairs judgment, promotes despair, and heightens dyscontrol, increases suicide risk. Yet, many persons with brain injury use illicit chemicals and abuse alcohol, placing themselves at even a greater risk for suicide.

Chemical abuse

Risk of damage associated with alcohol and drugs

Many persons with brain injury experience problems with chemical abuse. This includes the abuse of alcohol and the use of illicit drugs. This practice is problematic for a couple of reasons.

First, alcohol and drug use can affect cognitive functions.[12,13,14] Even when long-term changes have not occurred, their use affects immediate cognitive functioning. Alcohol use is a case in point. Few people, and certainly not those who abuse it, drink alcohol just for the taste; most people will admit that they have trained themselves to like the taste, and that their very first drink was often not a great taste experience. Alcohol is an acquired taste. The reason anyone uses such substances is because they change brain function. When one asks people why they use substances, the answers include the following: to forget problems, to fit in and decrease inhibitions (e.g., at a party), to help with depression, and to change perceptions. Memory (forgetting problems), executive functions (inhibition), emotional status (depression), and perceptual processing (change perceptions) are brain functions. If alcohol and illicit chemicals had no effect on the brain, people would not use them.

Since persons with brain injury already suffer from cognitive impairment, they can ill afford to incur further changes to their mental status. The world is a challenging place for most persons with brain injury: it is not easy to be successful, and most other people are not concerned about the needs of persons with brain injury. They are busy dating, working, running a business, etc. and have little consideration for the limitations of persons with brain injury. This is true even when persons with brain injury only have their original brain injury. When they add cognitive changes following chemical use, the hurdle they must overcome to succeed is likely to be too high. There are few people who care to help persons with brain injury to begin with, and there are even fewer willing to help people with brain injury compounded by further changes caused by substance abuse.

Another problem is that people who abuse alcohol and drugs have a lifestyle that places them at risk for further injury.[15] They have an increased probability of experiencing a second brain injury. Everyone recognizes the risks inherent in driving under the influence of alcohol or drugs. Less apparent, however, are the numerous other ways that the risk of brain injury increases with chemical use. People who are intoxicated or stoned may step off curbs and get hit by automobiles because they forget to look down the street or misperceive what they see. Drinking at a bar involves the risk of a fight, with a possible blow to the head. Drinking at sporting events also raises the chance of being in a fight. Illicit drug use entails drug purchases that incur the risk of brain injury — for instance, when a drug deal goes bad and one of the parties is hit over the head with a lead pipe (called being "piped"). In summary, if persons with brain injury persist in alcohol and drug use, the opportunity for additional damage to the brain increases due to these "indirect" risks.

The attraction and behavioral consequences of alcohol and drug use

Unfortunately, alcohol and drug abuse are tempting for persons with brain injury. They make them feel more sociable. They seem to make them feel less depressed. They can distort how well they believe they are doing.

With regard to alcohol, some persons with brain injury actually find that the place they seem to feel most "normal" and fit in best is at a bar. In a bar it is common to see people who are distracted and lose track of conversations. Many people are unable to remember what they are doing, and are forgetful. People in a bar may demonstrate slurred speech. With increasing consumption of alcohol, bar patrons begin to show balance problems. As inhibitions decrease, inappropriate social boundary violations occur. People in a bar can become aggressive. The evidence for the occurrence of aggression in a bar is the existence of a special term for it: a "bar fight." Going to a place where people are distractible and unable to remember things, lose track of conversations, show slurred speech, have trouble with balance, violate social boundaries, and participate in aggressive behavior may let some persons with brain injury blend in with other people.

Obviously, not all persons with brain injury abuse alcohol or drugs. Nevertheless, the risk is significant. Some persons with brain injury had their original injury because of alcohol use or drug abuse. It may have been a crucial precipitating element of the injury onset (e.g., drunken driving, falling downstairs, bar fight). Unfortunately, after their injury they continue their previous pattern of use. A second scenario occurs when persons with brain injury did not abuse alcohol or use drugs prior to onset and do not modify their alcohol use with injury, but their brain can no longer handle that unaltered level of use. Problems now develop despite no change in utilization. Finally, some people who had no problems before their injury now increase their alcohol use or initiate drug use, resulting in difficulties.

In summary, alcohol and chemical abuse can alter cognitive function. They also alter energy level and social skills. They distort emotional functioning. With all of these changes, it is not surprising that behavioral dyscontrol escalates. Behavioral dyscontrol accompanies emotional changes and cognitive deficits. Alterations in emotional and cognitive functioning, which alcohol abuse and drug use induce, increase the likelihood of behavioral dysfunction.

Persons with brain injury who are under the influence of alcohol or drugs show an increase in problem behaviors. Specific behaviors they may demonstrate include, for example, being less disposed to accept redirection. They may attempt to elope, and when thwarted become aggressive. They may become aggressive and then attempt to flee. Some become more isolative with alcohol and drug use. They withdraw socially, and their depression can increase. In contrast, they may show heightened activity but be socially inappropriate. They may say offensive things. They can violate social boundaries or be sexually inappropriate, reaching out and touching or grabbing other people.

Body image/pain/physical changes

Understanding the impact

Injuries that induce brain injury also cause physical impairments. The damage may be functional or cosmetic. Functional injuries include paralysis, spasticity, contractures, etc. Cosmetic changes include scars, disfigurements, hair growth pattern alterations, and so on. Some changes are both functional and cosmetic (e.g., cosmetic eyeball changes accompanying loss of vision). Some may be temporary, such as a shaven head after surgery. Nonetheless, even such temporary changes may be disturbing to persons with brain injury. For example, families who take pictures of loved ones, particularly of women with shaven heads, so that the persons with brain injury have a memento of the experience (like one might do after a broken leg with a cast), can inadvertently embarrass persons with brain injury, causing emotional trauma, because the family members do not understand the permanence of brain injury. Unfortunately, many changes after brain injury are permanent.

During hospitalization therapists routinely provide a strong focus on bettering physical limitations. The treatment can include improving physical abilities and instruction in compensation techniques. As part of this effort, therapists address emotional coping with alterations in physical skills. However, they generally pay less attention to physical disfigurement — scars, changes in hair growth patterns, distortions (even if subtle) in underlying bone structures, divergent eyes — which may not directly affect activities of daily living. After persons with brain injury are discharged from the hospital, their therapists and others with whom they come in contact may be even less mindful of the emotional impact of these changes. The emotional consequences can be quite significant.

Unfortunately, some persons with brain injury encounter not just benign neglect, but outright disregard of their feelings when they are told by others in response to their feelings about their physical appearance that they ought to focus on the "more important" outcome of their brain injury: namely cognitive problems leading to loss of friends, work, driving privileges, etc. This shortsighted diminishment of the emotional trauma associated with physical changes in appearance can infuriate persons with brain injury. While cognitive changes are intangible, changes in appearance are literally and figuratively "in your face." Even among the most self-actualized of individuals, such changes require considerable adjustment.

Coping with alterations in physical ability and appearance is hard. Physical evidence of an injury dissipates the ability of persons with brain injury to blend in; yet at the same time it may fail to elicit society's appreciation of the significance of the brain injury. This results in a lose–lose situation. It frustrates persons with brain injury, who also have an apparent physical disability, to have neither the advantage of being able to hide their injury nor that of receiving the assistance they need because of their brain injury.

One advantage that persons with brain injury who have no obvious physical disfigurement or impairment have over some other disability groups (e.g., persons with spinal cord injury) is that they can blend in when they want to fit into an environment. From outward appearances, no one knows they had a brain injury. Of course, the disadvantage of the lack of apparent injury that can be seen by the general population is that the injury seems less serious, and these persons with brain injury may receive much less help than they need. In contrast, persons with spinal cord injury theoretically receive the benefit of the doubt from people and can get help, although they sometimes receive more assistance than they desire. For example, persons with spinal cord injury may be ignored by waiters at restaurants, who inquire of their companions what the persons with spinal cord injury want to eat; it is difficult to hide a disability when one is in a wheelchair and the waiters forget that being unable to walk is different than being unable to talk.

A corollary problem for some persons with brain injury is overeating and weight gain. Some persons with brain injury experience significant weight gain. Weight gain may reflect brain injury-induced metabolic changes, or depression, boredom, and inactivity. The physical changes in appearance due to weight gain can have a negative impact on self-image.

The impact of all these types of physical change goes further than just image, however. Physical limitations can disrupt numerous life activities. The transformations in physical capabilities of persons with brain injury can be particularly devastating when they are already contemplating alterations in their life due to cognitive deficits. Imagine, for example, the frustration of coping with quadriplegia and life in a wheelchair while also having memory problems. It is difficult to utilize compensatory memory notebooks when they are kept behind the wheelchair in a pack that can be reached only by someone else. Moreover, the quadriplegia may interfere with an individual's writing ability. Perhaps this person's memory dysfunction leads to forgetting an appointment until the last minute, which cannot be compensated for by hurrying, due to physical limitations and balance problems. There are endless scenarios in which physical changes impair the ability of persons with brain injury to cope with cognitive difficulties.

Cognitive strengths normally help persons with physical disabilities address their challenges. Intelligence helps people outthink physical hurdles. Cognitive assets facilitate problem solving about barriers that physical limitations impose. There may be many alternative methods to accomplish a task, apart from the most common way, if one is smart enough and innovative enough to generate solutions. For persons who have both physical and cognitive impairments, however, the situation can be unbearable. Cognitive impairment limits problem solving about barriers that physical limitations impose, compromising the odds that persons with brain injury who have cognitive as well as physical difficulties will successfully determine and apply alternative compensation procedures.

An additional concern accompanying physical injury is chronic pain. Many persons with brain injury suffer from chronic pain. This includes posttraumatic headache.[16,17] Therapists might expect to see issues regarding pain in light of the extensive damage people incur when acquiring their brain injury and the physical forces involved in motor vehicle crashes and other onsets. However, health care providers tend to overlook pain or downplay its significance. This may result in part from providers' focus on the cognitive, behavioral, and emotional fallout of brain injury, which appear so overwhelming. Those concerns dominate the clinical picture. Pain, which cannot be seen or easily assessed, receives less attention. Furthermore, many rehabilitation therapists receive poor or no training in pain assessment and treatment. Parenthetically, there are efforts underway to treat pain as a vital sign in hospitals, to complement the current vital signs of temperature, pulse, blood pressure, and respiration.[18]

Pain care professionals, on the other hand, struggle to adopt their techniques to the needs of persons with brain injury. Persons with brain injury may lack the vocabulary and discriminative ability to precisely describe their pain. Cognitive impairment can interfere with vocabulary and cause language dysfunction, affecting the ability to make fine distinctions. For example, the McGill Pain Questionnaire[19,20] requires relatively sophisticated vocabulary to distinguish between word choices. Also, persons with brain injury respond differently to medications. They may have issues of medication noncompliance because of cognitive, behavioral, and emotional difficulties. Brain injury can also affect participation in chronic pain programs due to cognitive variables. Persons with brain injury may not remember information from a treatment group or may be unable to keep up with cognitively intact people who more quickly process the perspective that pain treatment therapists provide. Finally, if therapists consider persons with brain injury to be surgical candidates for pain amelioration, the question of the adequacy of cognitive processing gives rise to issues that range from the capacity to give informed consent to patients' expectations for a total cure of their pain. When therapists consider persons with pain for various treatments, they must evaluate the degree of fit between the pain treatment and the person with pain.[21] When candidates for pain treatment also have brain injuries, therapists must adjust treatment in light of brain injury considerations.

Behavioral dyscontrol

Physical injuries affect self-image, participation in life activities, weight, and pain level. The combination of physical injury and damage to cognitive processing compounds the harm that would be done by either alone. The impact of cognitive deficits and physical damage may lead to behavioral dyscontrol.

Persons with brain injury who feel distressed about how they look may demonstrate behavioral dyscontrol in reaction to society's response to their physical presentation. If people make comments about their appearance or show discomfort about being near them, persons with brain injury may react verbally or behaviorally. If other people shun them or ostracize them as a result of their outward physical features, then therapists should expect behavioral reactions. In extreme cases, persons with brain injury respond to the slights they feel by physically targeting those people they perceive to be unable to adjust to their appearance.

In other cases, the response may be more passive but just as significant. Some persons with brain injury may present as sad and depressed in response to physical changes. They may withdraw as a response to changes in appearance. Their appearance no longer fits in the range society defines as socially acceptable. As time passes and persons with brain injury become adept at physical compensation procedures, people dismiss the emotional scars of the physical changes. It seems that persons with brain injury who physically adapt to physical limitations are assumed to have adapted emotionally as well.

In fact, such an assumption is a fallacy and can lead to discharge from treatment before optimum adjustment has taken place. Unfortunately, financial pressures no longer allow the ideal time in treatment for persons with brain injury not only to learn physical compensation techniques, but also to accept them. In the past, the pace of treatment permitted acquisition of skills to match acceptance of their use. Sometimes this required months in treatment. It is important to understand that knowing how to do something does not necessarily mean wanting to do it or even being willing to do it. It certainly does not mean someone is going to do it. In the long run, rehospitalization can occur due to a failure to follow-through — that is, compliance — rather than because of inadequate instruction and skill acquisition. Inattention to issues of compliance causes difficulties. Persons with brain injury who fail to practice and apply physical adaptation techniques become more burdensome on their support system. Arguments leading to aggression easily erupt. Depression can result. Noncompliance increases. A decrease in compensation strategy utilization further limits relationships and socialization opportunities, and a downward cycle of behavioral dyscontrol ensues.

Issues of diet and weight gain can also cause behavioral problems. These issues often entail lack of acceptance of redirection about diet and access to food. Some persons with brain injury show little restraint regarding the consumption of large amounts of food or make poor nutritional choices. They may exceed their financial resources by selecting expensive food or too much food. Budget constraints may be a distant second consideration to the pleasure obtained through the immediate gratification received from eating. In hospital settings, therapists can observe inappropriate food selection in the hospital cafeteria. On outings, during activities outside of the hospital, problems of budgeting may arise at restaurants or in settings such as snack bars at zoos, malls, or movie theaters. At group homes, persons with brain injury may take food designated for a housemate. In any setting, persons with brain injury may hoard food. Therapist redirection about food selection, budgeting, and food possession frequently leads to inappropriate behavior. Outright aggression, deception, and denial are common responses.

Finally, pain causes irritability and poorer cognitive processing. It decreases tolerance of other people. Pain disrupts sleep. Persons with brain injury react to pain in the above manner much as do other people. However, with less cognitive, behavioral, and emotional resources, the likelihood for behavioral dyscontrol increases. Even among persons without brain injury who are in chronic pain, behavioral dyscontrol increases, with more anger, yelling, and fights. Brain injury exacerbates this dyscontrol.

Dating and sexuality

Introduction

Contrary to some peoples' beliefs about persons with disabilities, concerns about sex do not go away after onset of the injury. However, since sex is the issue therapists generally discuss least of all the challenges facing persons with brain injury,[22] it can become a major topic of concern. In fact, at support group meetings when persons with brain injury are given the opportunity to ask questions in an open-ended format, the two most common subjects are dating and sex. At conferences for persons with brain injury, the sessions on dating and sexuality draw some of the largest crowds.

Some persons with brain injury must cope with performance problems or physiological issues after brain injury.[23] As they would for anyone, such difficulties can cause distress, depression, isolation, and anger. It is part of the nature of brain injury that all aspects of human functioning can be affected. More common, however, are problems of psychosocial behavior as it relates to dating, relationships, and sex.

Problems selecting who to date

Persons with brain injury may lack the skills necessary to get a date and to date successfully. Dating is a complex behavior requiring knowledge, timing, and insight. To date successfully, persons with brain injury must start by selecting the correct people to approach for a date. All too often persons with brain injury select coworkers and therapists, including physicians, rehabilitation staff, transportation drivers, and group home providers. Their tendency to ask professionals for dates reflects their limited opportunities to meet other people. Moreover, the professionals on this list have a one-sided relationship with persons with brain injury. They frequently have intimate knowledge about persons with brain injury, but have not disclosed personal knowledge about themselves. To persons with brain injury they may seem ideal people for a relationship, since they are attentive to their needs without requiring anything in return. They solve problems and are caring without imposing any of their own problems or care needs on persons with brain injury. Hence, they are attractive and seem available.

Showing romantic interest in coworkers is a different problem. Many of these relationships fail, and the introduction of a dating relationship into a work environment is fraught with pitfalls. It is hard for anyone to avoid accusations of inappropriate behavior at work if entangled in a romantic situation. It is even more difficult for persons with brain injury to succeed at work while dating a coworker. Many persons with brain injury who attempt to initiate a dual relationship (i.e., coworker and date) are accused of harassment because their poor cognitive processing leads them to demonstrate their interest without regard for contextual cues, and they may be too intense or pursue their interest too long. When the relationship fails, persons with brain injury may face both an unsuccessful relationship and lost employment. Putting employment at risk to have a relationship with someone at work is unwise since many persons with brain injury struggle to find and keep a job. Jobs may last a long time, but budding relationships most often are temporary. It is injudicious to sacrifice a permanent job that was hard to obtain for a transient relationship. However, persons with brain injury may find this difficult to understand since they may observe uninjured coworkers initiating social relationships with their colleagues.

Problems with how to date

Assuming persons with brain injury select an appropriate potential date, they then face financial and logistical problems. Their economic status may limit activities. It is challenging to date on a limited budget. Part of dating is treating the other person to an activity, and that takes money. In addition, many persons with brain injury are unable to drive. Hence, getting to activities becomes a challenge. Public transportation hampers socializing and privacy. It is difficult for persons with brain injury to date when their home base is a group home or they are living with their parents. Such residences limit the opportunity for quiet, private time at home and may affect the perceptions the other person may have about dating someone with a brain injury.

Successful dating and relationships involve attending to the needs and desires of the other person. Many persons with brain injury find this difficult. Persons with brain injury must often monitor their own behavior to avoid dyscontrol, or at a minimum, inappropriateness. So much effort put into self-monitoring lessens the ability to appreciate the needs of a partner. As a result, persons with brain injury can seem self centered and egotistical. Moreover, because some persons with brain injury have limited social and recreational outlets, on a date they have little to share about themselves to help find common interests with a partner. Thus, they can seem one-dimensional and uninteresting. For example, since persons with brain injury are often unemployed, they have difficulty conversing about careers.

When persons with brain injury do get a date and they enjoy themselves, they frequently scare their partner away by being too intense about the relationship too quickly. If one has not had a date in a long time, the importance of the date and the value of the other person's interest can take on disproportionate significance. Love letters, flowers, and a request for second date the next day may chase away even people who have an interest in a second date.

Some persons with brain injury already have a partner and dating, per se, is not the issue. Instead, their problem is maintaining a relationship. Still, they face similar challenges regarding how to behave. Brain injury can affect intimacy skills,[24] whether in a dating situation or a long-term relationship.

Behavioral dyscontrol due to unsuccessful dating

Unsuccessful dating can lead to behavioral dysfunction. Whether the problem is due to selecting the wrong person, being too intense during or after a date, failing to notice the other person's needs during a date, lacking conversational topics and skills, or having insufficient money and transportation, the isolation and frustration that persons with brain injury experience can be the foundation for behavioral dyscontrol. Persons with brain injury may exhibit infatuation with therapists whom they have little chance of dating. Sometimes this can entail harmless fantasy. However, in some instances more serious issues develop. They may try to obtain personal information about therapists. Simple social questions can be probes to gather information about therapists' lives and families. Some persons with brain injury may begin to keep a list of therapists' names, the names of therapists' significant others, their phone numbers, etc. They may send therapists cards expressing affection, or even love letters. They may ask therapists on dates.

Persons with brain injury may direct their interest at popular culture figures. This type of infatuation may take an innocent form. They may hang up a commercially available poster of a celebrity. However, they may miss the social nuances of having a large poster of a scantily clad celebrity hanging on the wall when staff or visitors come to their rooms. In its most serious form, however, such adoration can manifest as delusional thought. Sometimes persons with brain injury believe that the celebrity has similar feelings for them. They may even believe that multiple celebrities share feelings for them at the same time or that an entire sports team would be willing to date them.

The risk to persons with brain injury of misguided efforts to establish a social or romantic relationship is one of frustration, depression, and anger at being rebuked and lost opportunities to establish real, enduring relationships. Becoming skillful at building relationships takes learning and practice. Wasteful efforts directed toward inappropriate targets of interest or affection increase social isolation. This enhances the problem of behavioral dysfunction.

Problems with sex

The same forces that interfere with dating can cause sexual isolation. Many persons with brain injury are sexually frustrated. Most people have fewer sexual encounters than dates, and so while some persons with brain injury may succeed at social relationships or dating, they may still be sexually isolated. Moreover, sexual performance can be more difficult than social performance. After all, even people without brain injury may struggle with the transition from a social relationship to one including sex.

Persons with brain injury may lack the skills necessary to transition a relationship to include sexual activity. Their word choice may be wrong or their timing may be off. They may misread the cues from the other person. Getting assistance in such skills is difficult and can even make therapists uncomfortable when persons with brain injury seek their instruction.

Moreover, as difficult as it can be to date, it can be even more difficult to perform well sexually. Persons with brain injury, hampered by potential difficulties with organically based divided attention and executive function problems, must attend to their partner's needs during a period of arousal and supreme distraction. All of the nuances of dating that persons with brain injury find so challenging are applicable during sex, but are multiplied by the intensity of the moment.

Behavioral dyscontrol due to issues of sex

Persons with brain injury can demonstrate behavioral dyscontrol based upon lack of sexual outlets or experiences of rejection or failure. Some seek physical contact in inappropriate ways. They may physically reach out to touch people on the genitals or breasts. At times such attempts may be obvious, but at other times persons with brain injury may mask their desires by apparent attempts at subterfuge, such as tilting back their head while in a wheel chair to rub the breasts of a female transport assistant. More blatant tries at sexual contact can occur. Some may try exposing themselves. They often explain their behavior by stating that because, for example, a therapist seemed to like them, they thought that exposing themselves would be viewed positively as an effort to reciprocate and initiate sex. Therapists may also experience outright offers of sex, such as when persons with brain injury are found naked in their rooms and explicitly offer to have intercourse with the therapists. Other persons with brain injury can be aggressive when seeking sex, and they may become assaultive.

Some persons with brain injury find sexual pleasure in masturbation. Difficulties befall them when they are indiscriminate as to time and place. In part, this is a "system" problem, as therapists may afford them little privacy in hospitals, nursing homes, or group homes. In addition, therapists, as well as persons with brain injury, may be uncomfortable discussing privacy in relationship to masturbation. Institutional rules may also be a problem. In many settings persons with brain injury have roommates or housemates with whom they must contend. However, persons with brain injury may contribute to their own difficulty when they fail to take into account time and place considerations. Society, represented by therapists and family members, tend to be unforgiving about errors in judgment regarding masturbation.

Persons with brain injury may seek sexual activity with prostitutes. Apart from the health risks to which anyone engaging in sex with prostitutes would be exposed, for persons with brain injury there are additional problems. They may be physically or financially abused as they seek sexual contact, because many persons with brain injury present to other people as vulnerable. They also risk running afoul of the law. Commonly, they lack legal resources and become afraid, having engaged in illicit activity with a poor conceptualization of the legal risks they are taking. If caught they may panic, becoming depressed and anxious. To find themselves in police custody, with cognitive impairment, is frightening and generates frantic calls to family or therapists. Police officers may offer deals based upon becoming a witness — a confusing turn of events if one is cognitively impaired, requiring set shifting, reasoning, judgment, and decision making in a short time while under pressure. Should such a negotiation take place, persons with brain injury face being witnesses with impaired memory, a daunting and possibly pointless exercise, that therapists can help persons with brain injury, police, and prosecuting lawyers avoid through helpful advice.

Many persons with brain injury do have consensual sexual partners. However, while this may remove some of the preceding hurdles to sexual outlet, it does not remove them all. Partners of persons with brain injury complain that issues of timing remain, as do considerations of the partners' sexual needs as persons with brain injury struggle with their own needs. Also, if persons with brain injury feel insecure as lovers, perhaps as a result of having experienced rejection from partners due to poor timing or the partners' depression and exhaustion from being both caregivers and the financial breadwinners, they may resent the time partners spend with friends — an escape from the task of caregiver at home, on one hand, and work, on the other hand. Jealousy easily becomes mistrust, or even paranoia, leading to accusations and outbursts. Innocent partners then become targets of aggression.

Lack of acknowledgment of deficits

The inability to perceive and acknowledge shortcomings is perhaps the most debilitating aspect of brain injury. While cognitive deficits may be a severe impairment to reentering life's activities, therapists can help address the worse cognitive impairments when persons with brain injury accurately recognize the problem. When limitations exist that persons with brain injury fail to take into account, the deficits can be insurmountable.

Lack of acknowledgment of difficulties primarily takes two major forms, though there can be variations[25] and, in truth, clinical presentations can be exceedingly complicated, reflecting the complex nature of brain processes that underlie awareness and acknowledgment of deficits.[26] Put simply, however, in the first form, persons with brain injury know something to be true about themselves, but it hurts too much emotionally to admit it is true. This type of denial is psychologically based, and persons with brain injury, as well as people in the general public without brain injury, engage in psychological denial. When people know that something is true about themselves but it contrasts with what they *want* to be true about themselves, they deny it is real. It is so painful to admit that they are not what they wish to be that they are unable to incorporate the truth into their view of themselves. For their own psychological health, they seek to ignore the truth about themselves or their actions. Persons with brain injury use psychological denial to protect their emotional functioning — and the existence of their self as a person — from the devastation of brain injury.

In the second form of lack of acknowledgment, in brief, persons with brain injury do *not* know the truth. This type of denial is organically based (i.e., "anosognosia," lack of awareness of deficits). Persons with brain injury experience organic denial because of the damage to the brain. Suppose someone breaks a leg. The uninjured brain, the examining instrument, adds up the data: "I cannot stand; I'm in pain; I am bleeding; my bone is sticking out through my flesh." The determination is, "I broke my leg." When the brain is damaged, it does not perceive the evidence: "my memory is fine; my reasoning is normal; I am concentrating well." The brain, the instrument that makes observations and determinations, is malfunctioning. It calculates and it gets the wrong answer.

Psychological and organic lack of acknowledgment of problems grossly interfere with the application of residual strengths and compensation for weaknesses, because persons with brain injury in denial are uninterested in investing in help. They are typically resistant to guidance and redirection. When they are determined to do something, they have lowered regard for the opinions of other people. Hence, they are noncompliant. They lash out at others who they judge to be unreasonably hindering their initiative.

Paranoia can develop from a combination of cognitive deficits and denial.[27] For example, imagine an event with ten bits of information, including the words said, tone of voice, setting, previous interactions, etc. A person with brain injury and a person without brain injury are present. The uninjured person attends to nine of the bits of information, understands eight, stores in memory seven, and recalls six. The person with a brain injury, being just slightly less efficient at each step, attends to eight of the bits of information, understands six, stores in memory four, and recalls two. After the event, the person with brain injury is angry, stating, "Joe (bit one) made fun of me (bit two)." The other person knows this, but also the following: it was at a party (bit three), the person with the brain injury made fun of Joe first (bit four), everyone was teasing each other (bit five), and Joe's comment was not intended to harm (bit six).

When told these additional bits of information, the person with brain injury does what everyone else naturally does: the person checks with the brain. "Did I forget something? Could that be true? Did I misperceive the situation?" The injured brain with memory deficits and reasoning problems is unable to locate any information on second review different than it first asserted: "No, Joe made fun of me." It does not have available additional information even upon second review.

In such situations, most people generally trust their own brain over the brains of other people, unless they locate information in their brain to support the other person's point of view. As with instant replay in football, unless "upon further review" there is incontrovertible evidence to the contrary, the decision stands: "Joe made fun of me."

When their view of events, people, and the world contradicts the perspectives of other people, persons with brain injury develop resentment and anger. It is easy to think: "I cannot be wrong all of the time. I must be right sometimes. Why is it that no one ever agrees with my viewpoint?" If there is an ongoing lack of consensual validation, mistrust arises. "If all of you think I am always wrong, then I no longer trust you. All of you are messing with me and are against me." In such circumstances, paranoid behavior develops and behavioral dyscontrol results.

Personality changes

Brain injury can change personality. The values, attitudes, interests, and perspectives on life of persons with brain injury may be different after the injury. This may reflect the emotionally traumatic, even near-death, experience of the brain injury onset. A conscious decision to reevaluate how one spends one's time plays a role. Moreover, cognitive impairment may direct the attention of persons with brain injury to different stimuli, changing how they view the world.

While therapists and families may hope that a new approach will be an improvement, this is not always the case. Some persons with brain injury become more self-centered or hedonistic. They may seek more immediate gratification. In exceptional cases, bigotry may be apparent where none existed before. (This is an atypical outcome; most persons with brain injury hope to use their experience to better themselves and help those around them.) However, when negative personality change occurs, behavioral dysfunction can be close behind.

Families are often quite distressed about the emergence of negative personality variables or even the resumption of previous, but unpleasant ones. Family relationships can be disrupted by the behavior of persons with brain injury who exhibit distasteful personality characteristics. In fact, early in rehabilitation, if personality tendencies that the family had hoped the brain injury might eliminate begin to reemerge, the families may come to therapists asking that whatever the therapists are doing that is causing the resumption of these previously present personality characteristics be stopped. They seek to have the premorbid negative traits "turned off." They may even bargain that they will accept more cognitive impairment in their loved one if less cognitive gain would correlate with less unwanted premorbid personality return.

Conclusions

Therapists who wish to change behavioral dysfunction must attend to the issues of adjustment that persons with brain injury confront every day. The challenges are broad and diverse, spanning every aspect of living, and continue throughout one's lifespan. Dealing with brain injury is a marathon. It is not a short haul or even a long haul. "It's a forever haul."[28]

There is no doubt that failure to adequately cope with the natural emotional consequences of brain injury impairs behavioral functioning. Part of establishing the appropriate neuropsychosocial environment involves the determination and appreciation of how issues of coping drive behavior.

References

1. *CARF 2001 Medical Rehabilitation Standards Manual*, Commission on Accreditation of Rehabilitation Facilities, Tucson, AZ, 2001.

2. Pflug, J. N., *Miles To Go Before I Sleep: My Grateful Journey Back From the Hijacking of Egypt Air Flight 648*, Hazelden, Center City, MN, 1996.
3. Osborn, C.L., *Over My Head: A Doctor's Own Story of Head Injury From the Inside Looking Out*, Andrews McMeel Publishing, Kansas City, MO, 1998.
4. Stoler, D.R. and Hill, B.A., *Coping with Mild Traumatic Brain Injury,* Avery Publishing Group, Garden City Park, N.Y., 1998.
5. Swanson, K.L., *I'll Carry the Fork: Recovering a Life After Brain Injury,* Rising Star Press, Los Altos, CA, 1999.
6. Carideo, A., Disability Insurance: Here's How to Find a Suitable Policy, *The Star Tribune*, Minneapolis, MN, May 13, 1987, 1M.
7. Stevens, M., Shop Carefully for Disability Insurance, *The Star Tribune*, Minneapolis, MN, October 19, 1987, 8M.
8. Beck, A.T., et al., *Cognitive Therapy of Depression*, Guilford Press, New York, 1979.
9. Blanchard, E.B. and Hickling, E.J., *After the Crash: Assessment and Treatment of Motor Vehicle Accident Survivors*, American Psychological Association, Washington, D.C., 1997.
10. Bongar, B., *The Suicidal Patient: Clinical and Legal Standards of Care*, American Psychological Association, Washington, D.C., 1991.
11. Karol, R.L. and Sparadeo, F., *Alcohol, Drugs, and Brain Injury,* Vinland Center, Loretto, MN, 1993.
12. Parsons, O.A., Alcohol abuse and alcoholism, in *Neuropsychology for Clinical Practice: Etiology, Assessment, and Treatment of Common Neurological Disorders*, Adams, R.L., et al., Eds., American Psychological Association, Washington, D.C., 1996, chap. 6.
13. Rourke, S.B. and Löberg, T., The neurobehavioral correlates of alcoholism, in *Neuropsychological Assessment of Neuropsychiatric Disorders*, Adams, K.M. and Grant, I., Eds., Oxford University Press, New York, 1996, chap. 18.
14. Wilson, J. T.L. and Wiedmann, K.D., Neuropsychological assessment in alcohol, drug abuse and toxic conditions, in *A Handbook of Neuropsychological Assessment*, Crawford, J. R., Parker, D.M., and McKinlay, W.W., Eds., Lawrence Erlbaum Associates, Hove, UK, 1992, chap. 15.
15. Gronwall, D., Wrightson, P., and Waddell, P., *Head Injury: The Facts*, 2nd ed., Oxford University Press, New York, 1998, chap. 7.
16. Packard, R.C., Epidemiology and pathogenesis of posttraumatic headaches, *J. Head Trauma Rehab.*, 14, 9, 1999.
17. Zasler, N.D., Posttraumatic headache: Caveats and controversies, *J. Head Trauma Rehab.*, 14, 1, 1999.
18. Pain Assessment and Management Standards, www.jcaho.org, Joint Commission on the Accreditation of Health Care Organizations, Accessed 11/20/02.
19. Melzack, R., The McGill pain questionnaire: Major properties and scoring methods, *Pain*, 1, 277, 1975.
20. Melzack, R. and Torgerson, W.S., On the language of pain, *Anesthesiology,* 34, 50, 1971.
21. Karol, R.L., Rehabilitation of the injured worker from a psychological perspective, in *Industrial Therapy,* Key, G.L., Ed., Mosby, New York, 1995, chap. 18.
22. Ducharme, S. and Gill, K.M., Sexual values, training, and professional roles, *J. Head Trauma Rehab.*, 5, 38, 1990.
23. Horn, L.J. and Zasler, N., Neuroanatomy and neurophysiology of sexual function, *J. Head Trauma Rehab.*, 5, 1, 1990.

24. Blackerby, W.F., Rediscovering intimacy, *TBI Challenge*, 1, 4, 1993.
25. Giacino, J. T. and Cicerone, K.D., Varieties of deficit unawareness after brain injury, *J. Head Trauma Rehab.*, 13, 1, 1998.
26. Prigatano, G.P. and Schacter, D.L., Eds., *Awareness of Deficit After Brain Injury*, Oxford University Press, New York, 1991.
27. Prigatano, G.P., O'Brien, K.P., and Klonoff, P.S. The clinical management of paranoid delusions in postacute traumatic brain-injured patients, *J. Head Trauma Rehab.*, 3, 23, 1988.
28. Sellars, C.W., Life care planning in catastrophic injury cases, presented at Minnesota Institute Legal Education Traumatic Brain Injuries Conference, Minneapolis, October 24, 2001.

chapter four

The phenomenology of behavioral dyscontrol

Conceptualization

Therapists must synthesize the information they gather about the cognitive and emotional functioning of each person they treat with brain injury into a conceptual framework of behavioral dyscontrol. Unprocessed raw cognitive and emotional data has little value until therapists organize it into clinical insights about the individual. The true impact of therapists who have experience working with behavioral dyscontrol after acquired brain injury arises from their skill in behavioral diagnosis: the ability to correctly conceptualize behavior. Behavioral planning requires therapists to accurately understand behavior and its determinants. Disjointed information about cognitive, emotional, and behavioral functioning cannot lead to successful treatment plans. Only through an appropriate formulation of behavioral determinants can therapists derive behavior plans that work.

The synthesis of information is very difficult in comparison to mere data collection on cognitive and emotional functioning. It is relatively easy to assess cognition using well-established procedures and tests, and many therapists are familiar with the determination of emotional status. However, organizing this information to develop a treatment plan is difficult. Therapists may focus on clinical observations but pull back when asked to formulate their view of the person with brain injury in a way that points to a treatment intervention. Experienced therapists are able to conceptualize behavioral dyscontrol in a manner that generates treatment interventions that work.

Correctly conceiving behavioral dyscontrol and creating appropriate treatment interventions requires clinical experience and confidence. Making observations is relatively simple, but developing a framework that a treatment team will follow for intervention in a given case exposes therapists' ideas to real-world corroboration or repudiation. This requires therapists to be willing to have their ideas tested by outcomes that will be observable by everyone.

In order to formulate behavioral plans, therapists need to understand the phenomenology of behavioral dyscontrol for each person with brain injury, or why, at a fundamental level, the person exhibits behavioral dyscontrol. The challenge for therapists is to discern and articulate this, and it will vary from person to person. A particularly important error occurs when therapists inadequately attend to antecedent conditions.[1] Erroneous conceptualization of the phenomenology of behavioral dyscontrol leads to a waste of time, resources, and money, because treatment will not be productive. Worse, persons with brain injury and their families will feel that there is no treatment that will work. This leads to hopelessness. Persons with brain injury may eventually be shunted to jail or state hospitals when it appears that therapists are incapable of developing a workable treatment plan.

The following sample scenario highlights the importance of therapists correctly recognizing the phenomenology of dyscontrol. Suppose therapists describe a person with brain injury as having "unprovoked aggression." This person reportedly has a history of hitting other treatment recipients or therapists "without any reason." The therapists who have worked with this person have been unable to identify antecedents to the behavior. Moreover, the cognitive functioning of this person is poorly understood. Emotional functioning is noted simply as "depression," "anxiety," or "anger." Hence, therapists make the attribution of "unprovoked aggression."

Consider how different the course of treatment might be with the correct determination of the phenomenology of this person's dyscontrol. Suppose that the cognitive assessment points to a very slow processing speed. This person demonstrates good receptive abilities and oral expressive skills that allow well-formed thoughts to be expressed, but typically after a long delay. Furthermore, history suggests that this person has little tendency toward verbal expression of emotions. Issues of self-image push the person towards individual action rather than teamwork. A sense of being right, with little tolerance of others, accompanies the person's rugged individualism. Finally, suppose this is a physically strong person who is used to intimidation of others and the application of force. This person now has organic damage increasing disinhibition.

Hence, our hypothetical person becomes annoyed by the perceived errors of others. Instead of seeking consultation with therapists, this person tries to figure out what to do without anyone's help. This person highly values being independent and self-reliant. Asking for help implies weakness, and since verbal expression of emotions is a little-practiced alternative, behavioral choices predominate. However, because it takes a while for the person to process observations, behavioral responses occur with little temporal relation to the annoyance. Nevertheless, adequate reasoning permits eventual development of a plan of action by the person.

Even when others quickly note irritability in this person, the lack of familiarity with expression of emotions, and the delay in articulating them, means that typically the person finds it easier and more comfortable to deny any concern than to make the effort to discuss the situation. Plus, the tendency toward individual problem solving suppresses dialogue. Therapists, even if they have noted something amiss, either do not ask the correct question to solicit a revealing response, fail to wait sufficiently long to accomodate slow processing speed, or become distracted by some other task or person. Then an hour later, or the next day, this person hits someone in an "unprovoked attack."

In reality, the aggression was not unprovoked. Rather, it was an understandable conclusion to a sequence of cognitive and emotional processing. Therapists with astute insight into the functioning of this person could have predicted the outcome. The phenomenology of dyscontrol for this individual includes the following elements: dislike of errors, belief in being right, inhibited verbal expression of emotions, valuing of machismo and individualism, problem solving through action rather than words, a long latency for cognitive processing, and use of physical strength.

Therapists' detection of the correct phenomenology of dyscontrol would lead to a well-formulated treatment plan for this individual, one not based on the idea that there is "unprovoked aggression." Rather, plan elements that take premorbid factors, current adjustment, and cognitive variables into consideration would address the behavioral dyscontrol. Of course, even experienced therapists may not get the phenomenology right the first time that they attempt a behavioral intervention. Some crucial variable in the history of a person with brain injury may be missing from the record or misunderstood. This hypothetical example is not intended to explain all cases of "unprovoked aggression," but rather to show one of many possible phenomenologies that might shed light on the etiology of such a case of behavioral dyscontrol.

Therapists should anticipate that coming to the correct phenomenological conceptualization of behavioral dyscontrol is very difficult. After all, if it were easy, everyone would get it right and there would be no problem with behavioral dyscontrol. Phenomenological conceptualization requires a knowledge base that encompasses clinical psychology, neuropsychology, neurology, psychiatry, nursing, physiatry, speech pathology, occupational therapy, physical therapy, social work, and so forth. Expertise in emotional adjustment, social history, family dynamics, behavioral management, cognitive functioning, neuropathology, physical functioning, etc. are necessary.

The development of a phenomenology of behavioral dyscontrol requires keen observation to apply the knowledge base mentioned above. Therapists will find clues to behavioral dyscontrol by being present when episodes occur. As trained observers with knowledge from the above fields of study already in place, skilled therapists will see explanations for behavior occurring before them. Such observations generate cognitive and emotional hypotheses to check against neurological data and behavioral, emotional, social, family, and organic history. Moreover, therapists who know this data before observing dyscontrol episodes can use these occurrences to confirm hypotheses they have generated from the data. Sometimes experimental scenarios may be devised to further generate and explore hypotheses.[2]

Therapists with experience in behavioral dyscontrol after acquired brain injury will "see" more than untrained observers will. Having a framework of academic and applied experience helps experienced therapists to notice things that less expert therapists miss or misinterpret. This is true in most fields of human endeavor: knowledge and experience count. It is certainly true in studying behavioral dyscontrol after acquired brain injury. Unfortunately, too often, behavioral plans are overly simplistic and poorly conceptualized because therapists did not avail themselves of a full understanding of everything going on with persons with brain injury.

Teams and rounds

Team models

To avoid insufficient phenomenological conceptualization, it is best for therapists to work in teams consisting of multiple disciplines. Therapists can maximize their grasp of behavioral dyscontrol by working in coordinated, integrated teams. First, therapists from different disciplines approach behavioral dyscontrol with diverse knowledge bases. Therapists from one discipline may notice or emphasize things that therapists from another discipline may miss or under-appreciate. Second, therapists from a variety of disciplines provide cross-fertilization. Different therapists might each have a piece of the total phenomenology, but until they join them together to compare ideas, each component may appear irrelevant or unimportant. The perspectives of one discipline based on therapists' knowledge and observations, taken in isolation, may not be enlightening until integrated with others' perspectives. Third, conversations with divergent disciplines lead to insights that none would have had alone.

It is important for therapists to correctly structure how the members of diverse disciplines will function in teams in order to maximize their success at conceptualizing behavioral dyscontrol. Multidisciplinary teams involve members of various disciplines who focus on their areas of expertise, but with little cross-fertilization. Interdisciplinary teams acknowledge overlapping areas of responsibility but still maintain exclusive control over core areas of responsibility. Supradisciplinary teams drop professional turf issues and acknowledge that all therapists can have input on any problem.[3] Supradisciplinary teams are the best model for the determination of the phenomenology of behavioral dyscontrol because they do not, *a priori*, assign particular problems to specific team members based on professional identification. Instead, this model opens up problem observation, solution generation, and treatment implementation to everyone on the team. The more brains assigned to a problem, the better.

Behavior rounds

It is also crucial for excellent care that there be frequent, routine meetings of all therapists working on a case for exploration of the phenomenology of dyscontrol. Of course, impromptu comparisons of thoughts on an immediate issue are also valuable, but these "hit and run" adjustments in behavioral plans cannot replace thorough exploration of the phenomenology of dyscontrol. Therapists must therefore schedule rounds to explore the phenomenology of dyscontrol on their cases. These "behavior rounds" go beyond traditional clinical rounds. In traditional medical rounds, therapists report patient progress. However, while there may be an exchange of information, time constraints and the structure of these meetings usually are not conducive to freewheeling concept generation and problem solving. In contrasting these traditional medical rounds with the creative behavior rounds described in this chapter, imagine the difference between a meeting where an advertising agency presents an advertising product to a client versus the back room free-for-all meetings early in the development stage.

Behavior rounds work best when they are somewhat unstructured. Therapists need to feel encouraged to voice their observations and conceptualizations. Such behavior rounds are a requirement for open discussion of behavioral problems.[4] Behavior rounds are an opportunity to compare perspectives and, perhaps most importantly, for therapists to disagree with one another. Therapists often derive their best ideas after respectful disagreements. Appreciation of the phenomenology of dyscontrol for each person with brain injury takes time to form, and there can be false starts along the way. Experienced therapists may not obtain unanimity in their perspectives on the phenomenology of dyscontrol, particularly early in case conceptualization. However, successful intervention does require two aspects of team functioning, described below, when unanimity escapes the team.

First, when the team of therapists disagrees it must be done with respect. This should be obvious, but teams have disintegrated when therapists forget that it is their *idea* that is at issue, not themselves as people or professionals. Therapists may experience a stretch of time when their ideas are challenged. However, they create a poor environment for treatment when they connect their personal or professional egos to other therapists' agreement with their ideas. Therapists who resent others whose ideas conflict with their own can become hostile, or worse, passive-aggressive. The destructiveness of such therapists on the morale of other therapists, team effectiveness, and the eventual application of a neuropsychosocial environment is inestimable. It is essential that therapists working to devise and implement neuropsychosocial environments have a strong sense of professional self-assurance and can handle having their ideas rejected.

Second, despite spirited disagreements about the phenomenology of behavioral dyscontrol for a person with brain injury, when the team settles on a neuropsychosocial environment to create, all of the therapists must fully commit to its implementation, even if it might not be founded on the phenomenological conceptualization every therapist proposed or the neuropsychosocial environment they supported. To give a fair trial of successful implementation, all of the therapists must pull together to create the agreed-upon neuropsychosocial environment. The therapists may later determine that, in fact, they selected an incomplete, inadequate, or wrong phenomenology in their initial planning or that a different neuropsychosocial environment is required for success, either as an adjunct to or replacement of the original. If so, returning to an idea previously proposed by a therapist is not a reflection of the blinding wisdom of that therapist or the poor abilities of the therapists who initially pushed for the less than totally successful ideas that were adapted, but rather is evidence of the difficulty in treating severe behavioral dyscontrol after acquired brain injury. All therapists will have their turn at having the team try their ideas, at being right and wrong prospectively and retrospectively.

To participate in behavior rounds, therapists must be able to think outside of the box. The purpose of behavior rounds is to generate ideas about the phenomenology of behavioral dyscontrol and the neuropsychosocial environment. These cannot occur through adherence to dogma about behavioral etiology or intervention. Rather, therapists must be innovative. Effective generation of ideas requires an initial stage during which therapists produce thoughts for the next step of selection. In this first stage, therapists should be encouraged to play with ideas. Some reflections may be considered impractical upon further consideration. Others may seem unethical or otherwise objectionable after more reflection. Sometimes therapists determine that a suggestion about a component of the neuropsychosocial environment is too tangential to the phenomenological understanding of the person with brain injury to be effective. Nevertheless, a freewheeling exchange of theses and rationales is essential for the development of the phenomenology of dyscontrol and the creation of a neuropsychosocial environment.

Finally, behavior rounds can also serve as an informal support group for therapists. Therapists may express feelings of being afraid of particular persons with brain injury. They may raise concern that a particular treatment plan is too risky. Therapists may become angry with certain persons with brain injury, or they may find some behaviors to be personally repulsive. Therapists may express ethical or moral concerns about treatment ideas. A wise group of therapists will recognize these thoughts and feelings as a reflection of the difficult work in which they are engaged and of the commitment to excellence that the therapists have. Inexperienced teams will find such anxieties to be a distraction, whereas knowledgeable therapists will know that support for such openness bonds teams together, a prerequisite for a coordinated neuropsychosocial environment and a stellar treatment outcome.

Phenomenological variables

There are too many possible formulations for behavioral dyscontrol that therapists might devise to list them all here. Most real life formulations are exceedingly complex, as will be seen in Chapter 8, which provides clinical vignettes. As a prelude to that chapter, the following pages provide some basic considerations, albeit with some trepidation. They represent some starting points to help move therapists from data collection to treatment planning; they are not a "cookbook" for treatment plans. Therapists will encounter other crucial variables, and those provided here are likely to be much more complicated when seen in the real world.

Dependency

Many persons with brain injury exhibit behavioral dyscontrol as a result of their sense of dependency. One hallmark of brain injury is the need for assistance in at least some areas of life: activities of daily living (ADL), transportation, housing arrangements, employment, and legal and financial decision making. Persons with brain injury rebel as therapists, families, employers, and lawyers intrude on their sense of independence. After all, most people devote the first twenty plus years of their lives to gaining their independence (and probably the last years of their lives fighting to maintain it). People do not readily sacrifice their independence. So when brain injury threatens their independence, persons with brain injury fight against those who threaten to remove it.

Therapists can observe resistance to dependency for small, brief activities as well as large, sweeping ones. Persons with brain injury may hit, kick, spit, or throw things at therapists during therapists' assistance with dressing, toileting, or getting in or out of bed, even when the person with brain injury wants the activity to be completed. It would seem to a casual observer that this is a strange moment to be aggressive considering that the person with brain injury and the therapist agree on the completion of the activity. However, the sense of dependency, loss of control, and perhaps the feeling of shame in needing help with basic activities can lead to aggression. Sometimes the person needs help and hates it. At other times, it is an opportunity to exert control. When persons with brain injury resist direction they may gain a sense of mastery over their own fate. Certainly, should therapists and the person with brain injury disagree about the provision of assistance, either as to its timing, type, or its need at all, the potential for behavioral dyscontrol escalates. Therapists may, in fact, see dyscontrol resulting from seemingly trivial directions, where the sense of dependency on the part of persons with brain injury is the hidden phenomenological variable.

More wide-ranging examples also exist. Removal of driving privileges frequently results in noncompliance. Persons with brain injury after hospital discharge ask most often for a return of the privilege to drive. Sometimes they are more persistent in asking therapists about driving than about being allowed to return to work. The acquisition of driving privileges in teenage years represents a rite of passage. It is a statement of being on the threshold of adulthood, and in reality, provides geographic emancipation: one can move around independently. It is almost as good as the freedom one obtains by learning to walk. Persons with brain injury do not suffer the removal of such independence lightly. They fight back: they steal keys; they drive without permission. They physically assault family members who try to stop them from driving. They refuse to visit therapists who provide data against their driving.

Prohibitions against return to work because of brain injury also induce a sense of dependency. Holding a job represents more than financial security. When brain injury truncates employment, persons with brain injury can become isolated. They are unable to take advantage of the possibilities work offers for the establishment of friendships. They are not present for social activities that work provides: Friday after-work gatherings, holiday parties, small group gatherings, and so on. In addition, they typically have less money to spend on social and recreational pursuits. This limitation again isolates them. Persons with brain injury who cannot work miss the feeling of satisfaction that accompanies returning something to society. Productivity breeds wellbeing. Guilt develops when persons with brain injury are always on the receiving end of exchanges with other people and society. Self worth declines.

Awareness by persons with brain injury that they are more dependent than other people leads to behavioral dyscontrol. Dependency causes shame, guilt, poor self-esteem, and then anger. Attempts by therapists during rehabilitation to encourage awareness of deficits so that reasonable treatment planning can proceed may backfire as therapists encounter resistance, and perhaps aggression, during the early stage of delineating limitations prior to treatment. Furthermore, when therapists work with persons with brain injury during transition to home, group home, or nursing home or when they try to help with return to work, driving, financial planning, etc., and offer educational information regarding strengths and weaknesses, they may see an increase in anger and noncompliance because the persons with brain injury readily perceive the implications of limitations for personal, financial, social, and recreational accomplishment. Angry, isolated, guilty people rarely demonstrate a calm, reflective demeanor. Further behavioral problems are the usual corollary of such emotions. Chapter 7 presents further perspectives on the sense of dependency and how therapists might re-conceptualize it for persons with brain injury

In summary, one crucial variable to consider when therapists conceptualize the phenomenology of dyscontrol is dependency. Dependency may give rise to numerous expressions of behavioral problems.

Privacy

Persons with brain injury often lack privacy. Privacy provides time to think for problem solving, reflection upon events that have occurred, and contemplation of hopes for the future. When persons with brain injury are deprived of privacy, behavioral dyscontrol escalates.

Consider the effect of living arrangements on privacy. In some hospital settings persons with brain injury may live in double rooms. As they must cope with the most severe of injuries — brain injury — they are faced with a roommate they do not know. The roommates' friends and family visit, intruding on privacy. The difficulties that the person with brain injury must work to ameliorate become the public knowledge of the roommate and the accompanying family and friends, all strangers. The assistance the person with brain injury now requires is observable by people they have never met before their injury.

Even if persons with brain injury are fortunate enough to have a single room, the threat to privacy does not dissipate. Therapists are continually entering their room, sometimes even intruding on bathroom activities, care being offered by other therapists, or intimate moments with family. Therapists are usually trained to knock before entering, but over time therapists may become casual about this, either performing a perfunctory knock or omitting it altogether. Sometimes therapists do knock, appropriately, but then fail to wait for a reply, entering before really receiving permission.

Even when therapists are diligent about respecting privacy, the *sense* of privacy may be tenuous. Privacy encompasses two elements: being left alone and knowing one will be left alone. While knocking on doors before entering is helpful for signaling that therapists intend to enter, persons with brain injury know that a knock can come at any time. True privacy includes the knowledge that no one will, or even can, be a disturbance: it is only when one is so secure that a real sense of privacy exists and true relaxation is possible. Contemplate the sense of privacy and ease people feel when they are in their own homes behind locked doors. In hospital settings, persons with brain injury are not permitted to have a lock on their door. If therapists knock on the door and then really wait for permission to enter, persons with brain injury who withhold permission too long find therapists entering to find out "what is wrong."

Similarly, privacy is missing in nursing homes. The same issues exist, though likely worse because single rooms are considerably more rare in nursing homes than in hospitals. In addition, extended nursing home stays may increase therapists' familiarity with persons with brain injury, subsequently increasing a casual attitude toward privacy. Therapists may assume a relaxed perspective towards privacy naturally accompanies familiarity but fail to inquire from the persons with brain injury as to whether they agree. When asking what privacy restrictions persons with brain injury desire, therapists must remain aware, also, that persons with brain injury may acquiesce to therapists' suggestions without really wanting to implement them. This happens because persons with brain injury may feel they will displease or offend therapists when they want greater privacy protections than therapists feel are necessary. Persons with brain injury who are dependent on therapists may feel uncomfortable insisting on privacy restrictions.

Theoretically, group homes ought to offer privacy beyond that seen in hospitals and nursing homes. After all, a group home is a house, commonly with only four persons with brain injury living together. Nevertheless, to those living there it hardly seems like what they may have contemplated as their dream home. Few people envision living with four strangers monitored by rotating staff as their eventual permanent living arrangement. Group homes also put privacy at risk in manners similar to hospitals and nursing homes, but they may compromise privacy in unique ways. Hospitals and nursing homes may provide a semblance of privacy due to their larger size, which offers anonymity. Not everyone in a hospital or nursing home knows who a particular person with brain injury is. Not even everyone on a particular floor or ward may know everyone. However, group homes are more intimate. Everyone knows everyone. Everyone tends to see everything that happens, in part because many of the occurrences affect everyone in the home. Therapists know everyone when there are only four residents. Families of housemates may also become familiar with each other and with all four persons with brain injury living in the group home.

Of course, there is an advantage to familiarity. In hospitals it is desirable to have therapists who frequently check on persons with brain injury. Medical care requires entering rooms, sometimes even when one wants to be left alone. Similarly, in nursing homes, persons with brain injury may wish to restrict access against their own best interests. A sense of shared interest, concern for and a desire to help each other, and familiarity with housemates makes group homes attractive. Problems arise when therapists and persons with brain injury disagree about the balance between good care and privacy.

At work, privacy problems may also develop. Coworkers may find out about a person's unapparent brain injury. In other cases the injury may be readily apparent. Supervisors may be indiscreet when handling issues related to persons with a brain injury. The presence of job coaches compromises privacy.

Transportation challenges privacy. Because many persons with brain injury are unable to drive, they depend on others for travel. Sometimes this requires family or friends to transport them. There are two ways in which this interferes with privacy. First, it means that the driver knows about all the activities of the person with a brain injury. This may involve business dealings or social engagements. Dating, for example, is difficult when a third party drives. Second, for many uninjured people, time spent driving is private time away from other people. This is lost if someone else must drive the person with a brain injury.

A common alternative is publicly paid transportation for persons with disabilities. Persons with disabilities, including brain injury, can call in advance to arrange a ride. However, transportation services provide these rides in vans with the name of the service prominently displayed, declaring to the world that the people entering or exiting the vans have disabilities. Persons with brain injury, or others with disabilities, are unable to use such a van discreetly. Furthermore, these vans accommodate multiple individuals, further reducing privacy. Finally, van drivers can sometimes be insensitive to the privacy preferences of the persons they serve.

People have a need at times to be left alone and to have thoughts, feelings, or actions that they withhold from general public observance. They may choose to share their time and private lives with the public, or in a more limited fashion, with close friends or family. It can be infuriating when persons with brain injury are exposed by their disability to intrusions on their privacy contrary to their wishes. A wide range of behavioral dyscontrol can occur when privacy is threatened. Persons with brain injury may resist participation in activities, preferring to be alone. They may sabotage prerequisite planning. They may be passive–aggressive, for example, getting ready too slowly, so as to disrupt the preparation for an event. They can even barricade themselves in their room. Attempts by therapists to encourage them to join in activities may backfire. Depression and anger may increase. Persons with brain injury may direct physical aggression at those who fail to respond to their less blatant attempts to deflect participation.

Behavioral dyscontrol can also arise when privacy violations happen in a less apparent manner than through enforced participation in activities. A single invasion of privacy may trigger an outburst if it occurs at an inopportune moment. Certainly, repeated violations of privacy can destroy trust, the foundation of an enduring therapeutic relationship. Persons with brain injury determine with whom they feel most at ease. When rapport exists with therapists, persons with brain injury are more likely to comply with requests and directives than when they are suspicious of the therapists. When therapists honor privacy concerns, they build a base upon which to establish rapport and trust, the prerequisites for a caring, successful, therapeutic relationship that decreases episodes of behavioral dyscontrol. It is therefore important that therapists weigh the impact that loss of privacy has upon behavioral dyscontrol. Understanding the phenomenology of dyscontrol for many persons with brain injury requires contemplation of issues of privacy.

Scheduling

Freedom to establish one's own schedule is an important aspect of control over one's life. Persons with brain injury often lose their freedom to set their own schedules. They can be dependent upon the desires of others for their schedules. Brain injury can ruin the freedom people typically have to select their own schedules for various reasons. Sometimes loss of control of schedule results from being dependent on other people for transportation. If others must drive persons with brain injury, the schedule of the drivers becomes a factor. This is true whether the schedule of the drivers is personal, as in the case of family or friends, or corporate, as in the case of public van transport services. In the latter instance, for example, persons with brain injury are restricted to the hours of operation of the transportation service.

Persons with brain injury may lose control of their schedules because of cognitive problems. To set up and manage appointments takes considerable cognitive acumen. One must know how close together one can program various appointments and commitments. It is crucial to factor in the whims of others in one's schedule: the likelihood of their being on time, their reliability in keeping appointments, their efficiency during activities so that an appointment or task ends on time, etc. Next, one must be flexible in reconfiguring one's schedule as situations change. Adaptability and skill in redesign can relieve much distress. Finally, one must remember one's schedule either through excellent memory or dedicated utilization of calendars, appointment books, or hand-held computer devices. Thus, scheduling requires insight into the threats others pose to one's schedule, adaptability and tolerance for change, and memory functioning. Insight, adaptability, and memory may be lacking after brain injury.

Persons with brain injury who mis-schedule, exhibit rigidity, or forget appointments or activities lose control of their schedules. Other people take charge setting up where they are supposed to be and when they are supposed to be there. Other people establish with whom persons with brain injury are to meet. For example, persons with brain injury get little input into their treatment schedule, selection of therapists, order or frequency of cares, and so forth. People without cognitive deficits are better able to assert their preferences. Such individuals can advocate more effectively for their own interests than can persons with brain injury.

Persons with brain injury can become very irritated with the loss of input into their schedules. Continually being vulnerable to the preferences of other people is frustrating. Persons with brain injury may react to this with behavioral dyscontrol. Such behavioral dyscontrol takes many forms. Persons with brain injury may show verbal aggression, including anger in response to schedule changes. Threats can ensue when they are unable to set their schedules as they desire. Outright harassment of others may result: for example, they may disrupt physician offices through intimidation.

When persons with brain injury make errors in their schedules, they may lash out at other people, blaming them for mistakes they made themselves. If they forget to record an entry in an appointment book, they may accuse someone else of not telling them about the appointment. If they are late and the people they were to meet no longer can devote sufficient time to their issues, they become angry with the other people. They may accuse others of disinterest.

When other people step in to provide help with scheduling to persons with brain injury, they may encounter resistance. Persons with brain injury may view their help as interference. Persons with brain injury may actively resist help through aggression or they may use subterfuge. They may hide appointments from concerned family or friends. They may cancel appointments other people have scheduled for them, or they may just not appear for the appointment. Alternatively, they may attend an appointment, but be uncooperative during the appointment.

In summary, issues of scheduling control can easily lead to behavioral dyscontrol. Scheduling is a process that many uninjured people take for granted. Few people are aware of the significance persons with brain injury place on input into their schedule. Inability to dictate their schedule has far-reaching emotional consequences that can underlie behavioral problems. Wise therapists should consider the impact loss of scheduling control has on persons with brain injury as they develop the phenomenology of behavioral dyscontrol for each person.

Goal setting

Human beings feel best when they can set their own goals. A distinguishing characteristic of adulthood is the freedom people have to establish what future they want to work towards. Children have goals set for them by adults. For example, children are told they must go to school, and parents set expectations for what they will consider to be satisfactory achievement levels. Parents filter recreational pursuits, determining the nature and frequency of social engagements and activities.

As independent adults, people get to choose their own goals. Society permits adults to set high standards or low ones for themselves. This is not so for many persons with brain injury. Persons with brain injury frequently are told what goals they ought to have. Moreover, therapists are taught to help maximize treatment outcomes. Woe be to persons with brain injury who state that they have had enough therapy and are satisfied with their achievement, if the treatment team believes they can accomplish more. When persons with brain injury beg off, declaring that enough is enough, a whole treatment bureaucracy engages to persuade them of the value of greater achievement. This ranges from therapists to facilitate motivation to insurance companies who question malingering. It is antithetical to our health care values that those receiving care might not wish to make use of everything that can be made available. Thus, persons with brain injury lose the right to say no.

Persons with brain injury ought to be encouraged to avail themselves of all our treatment system can provide. It would be unethical to fail to offer care that might help them. It would, moreover, be wrong to withhold assistance that would help them maintain motivation, particularly during periods of frustration and depression. Furthermore, premature termination requests due to lack of awareness or acknowledgement of deficits ought not to be indiscriminately granted. Nevertheless, a balance must be struck between support, encouragement, and facilitation of treatment and ignoring the wishes of persons with brain injury. When therapists wrest control of goal setting from persons with brain injury, behavioral dyscontrol appears. For many persons with brain injury, this feels like a return to childhood. In response to decreased determination of their own goals, they rebel. Therapists may see noncompliance, aggression, and sabotage of treatment.

The problem of goal setting extends beyond just treatment environments. In group homes, where there is recognition of the importance of behavioral management, therapists work on goals with persons with brain injury keeping the views of these persons in mind while being cognizant of behavioral management concerns. In contrast, in group homes where there is inexperience with behavioral management after brain injury, therapists tend to set expectations and goals without regard to the abilities or desires of persons with brain injury. Therapists then express astonishment when behavioral difficulties escalate, but rarely do they acknowledge their own contribution to the problem.

A common example demonstrates this remarkably well. Group homes will admit persons with brain injury with plans to have them attend a day program. Such planning occurs without consideration of whether persons with brain injury *want* to go to the day program, to say nothing about the match of the day program with the needs of persons with brain injury, the capability to arise on time and meet the day program schedule, or the difficulties transportation engenders. Of course, these issues may have a significant impact in the determination of whether persons with brain injury want to go to the day program, but it may also be possible that some other pursuit is more attractive, perhaps even just staying at home. The issue is not whether the alternatives persons with brain injury advocate for are reasonable; but whether therapists consider the choices persons with brain injury put forth, and, if impractical, how they address the feelings they will have about being thwarted in their hopes. Unless therapists attend to the goals persons with brain injury want to work toward, they will encounter behavioral dyscontrol.

Therapists also set vocational goals for persons with brain injury. Many persons with brain injury held jobs prior to onset or at least were in school pursuing training for vocational interests. Certainly most, except the very young, had some vocational aspirations. Now, after their brain injury, therapists direct them to particular career activities. They encounter a team of therapists, including physicians, neuropsychologists, occupational therapists, vocational counselors, job coaches, etc., who voice opinions on return to school or work. Persons with brain injury cannot ignore these opinions as if they were casual advice. These therapists in essence are gatekeepers who control needed approvals before employers will permit return to work or will complete a fresh hire. Furthermore, governmental bodies establish regulations about earning ceilings above which persons with brain injury lose disability support. Persons with brain injury must therefore incorporate salary cap considerations in job pursuits so that return to work does not decrease income or benefits.

People without injuries obviously function differently. While they may seek advice, they are free to choose their education and work. Most people conceptualize salary as "the more, the better." In a capitalistic democracy, freedom to choose work is an accepted right, a basic tenet of the system. Persons with brain injury see this right truncated and they rebel. They may become noncompliant, not just with vocational guidance, but with other matters as well, when resistance due to frustration contaminates other decision making. If poor vocational choices lead to failure, then financial resources may be squandered, causing additional stress and inappropriate behavior. Depression due to alterations in self-esteem, founded on the link between job and self-image, may worsen behavior. Blocked vocational desires can be the most devastating of consequences from brain injury, often causing the most resistance to redirection due to poor insight and struggles with acceptance.

Therapists with expertise in behavioral dyscontrol will reflect upon the contributions of lost goal setting to the phenomenology of dyscontrol. They can address much behavioral dyscontrol by paying attention in behavioral planning to the desire of the person with brain injury to be involved in goal setting.

Physical status

Many persons with brain injury experience inappropriate levels of physical activity. For some, there is too little activity. Their injury may limit the nature of the activities in which they can participate. For example, bicycle riding may be impossible for those who use an electric wheelchair for mobility. For other persons with brain injury who could otherwise ride a bicycle, balance problems may be prohibitive. Additional limitations such as problems with coordination, motor speed, visual-spatial disturbances, etc. may interfere with physical recreational pursuits unless modifications are available. However, persons with brain injury frequently encounter resistance from other people to necessary modifications because other people find the changes inconvenient or expensive, or they feel that some enhancements might give persons with brain injury an advantage during competition (e.g., equipment that enhances performance).

Financial concerns are another hurdle to involvement in customary physical activities. Participation in sports frequently entails expenditures. Teams and leagues may require fees. Equipment may be expensive. Health club memberships can be costly and are not typically designed for people with special needs. For example, health club swimming pools are not generally wheelchair accessible.

When people are inactive, physical discomfort increases. Boredom may be another side effect of inadequate physical activity. Insufficient daily energy expenditures may alter sleep. When persons with brain injury are physically inactive, as with anyone else, they may become uncomfortable, tired, and ill at ease. Finally, a person's sense of well being may decline without physical activity, which may result in escalation in behavioral dyscontrol.

For other persons with brain injury, the completion of their daily routine requires so much effort that they experience continual periods of fatigue. Activities that uninjured people complete without a second thought may require substantial cognitive and physical effort on the part of persons with brain injury. Such individuals are indulging in too much consumption of physical energy and become drained. They tire easily. Tired people are more irritable. Thus, activity can also prove to be a source of behavioral dyscontrol.

In addition to too little or too much physical activity, pain, regardless of activity level, can be a significant source of behavioral dyscontrol. People in persistent pain tend to have fewer emotional reserves and may be less tolerant. They may exhibit more annoyance at people and events. Consequently, persons with brain injury who are in pain have a greater likelihood of behavioral dyscontrol.

Therefore, therapists must consider the impact of inappropriate physical activity or pain on expressions of behavioral dyscontrol. Too often, therapists miss these factors, since a particular activity level is treated as just part of the person's basal presentation, like height or hair color. However, knowledgeable therapists consider activity level as something imposed by the environment that they can alter. Such therapists evaluate physical activity as part of the phenomenology of behavioral dyscontrol.

Sexual isolation

Therapists should avoid underestimating the impact sexual frustration can have on behavioral dyscontrol. The range of behaviors that therapists observe is limitless. Some examples include:

- Inappropriate comments about other people's appearance (comments which are too intimate, said in the wrong setting, at the wrong time, in the wrong tone of voice, or with the wrong accompanying facial expression, body language, or gesture)
- Touching inappropriately (in the wrong setting or time, with the wrong person, or too intimately)
- Grabbing (particularly the wrong body part, but also not releasing a handshake in the socially acceptable time frame, trying to stroke the hand slightly, or just relishing the contact of the other person's hand too much)
- Making sexually implicit or explicit comments (offering sex, requesting sex, using rude language in a conversation in an attempt to invite similar language and establish a perceived bond)
- Exposing body parts (pulling down pants, throwing off bed covers while wearing insufficient or no clothes, stroking one's own body parts to solicit contact)

The behavior can range from subtle — leaning back into a therapist's breast while in a wheelchair during transport — to overt, such as going to a prostitute.

It is easy for most therapists to hypothesize underlying issues of a sexual or social nature when the behavior is sexually tinged. However, experienced therapists know that the effect of sexual isolation can also drive behaviors that are not sexual in presentation, such as generalized noncompliance or aggression. Knowledgeable therapists will attend to the possibility of sexual issues underpinning diverse behaviors. Therapists place behavioral programming at risk when they omit the potential contribution of sexual isolation from the phenomenology of behavioral dyscontrol.

Emotional incontinence

Brain injury can cause unintended emotional states. Persons with brain injury may be unable to inhibit swings in emotions. These emotional changes may be unrelated to particular events or they may be exaggerated emotional responses to events or people. Behavioral programming must consider the degree to which emotional presentations reflect intentional feelings versus uncontrollable affect or mood. When emotions are out of control, behavioral dyscontrol can quickly follow. The inability of some persons with brain injury to establish their affect or mood gives rise to many of the behavioral problems therapists encounter.

Behavioral difficulties that occur due to excessive emotionality are the most common problem. Lowered mood typically leads to less severe problems, though it may contribute to lack of initiation problems. Persons with brain injury who become unstable with or without provocation and overshoot the degree of appropriate anger and hostility present a significant risk for behavioral dyscontrol. However, even excessive happiness, an admittedly strange concept, can lead to behavioral problems when persons with brain injury cannot control excitement. Some persons with brain injury, upon receiving good news, become literally overjoyed. They cannot attend to task. They are preoccupied with or even perseverative about the information. They may become overly aroused. Sleep can be disrupted. Hence, from a state of exuberance comes an inability to accept direction; arousal becomes intolerance; sleep deprivation triggers irritability.

A case in point would be persons with brain injury who cannot handle praise without losing control. Some persons with brain injury lose their willingness to listen to advice or instructions when they receive feedback on how well they are doing. They become headstrong and their compliance disintegrates. A related example can be seen when persons with brain injury anticipate a team meeting in which they expect positive things to be discussed. In anticipation of the meeting they may become overexcited, and this excitement spills over into lack of redirectability because of arousal. Hence, it is important for therapists to contemplate the effect uncontrolled emotional changes have on behavior. Knowledgeable therapists consider emotional incontinence involving both positive and negative emotions when formulating the phenomenology of behavioral dyscontrol.

Grief

Most persons with brain injury experience grief. They have a significant sense of loss. Sometimes this involves loss of work or relationships. It may entail loss of other things that are important to them: living arrangements, recreational activities, or money. Usually the loss also includes a generalized sense of having lost one's abilities across the spectrum of skills. Particularly early after onset (a few months to a year, but sometimes for years) persons with brain injury may describe a pervasive feeling of loss unlinked to any specific losses. Grief is a powerful emotion and can lead to behavioral dyscontrol in the form of noncompliance or more active aggression when therapists pressure them to be more active in rehabilitation while they only want to withdraw and grieve their losses.

Grief also arises when persons with brain injury lose their emotional support system. Sometimes this is the direct result of the onset: for example, when people important to the person with brain injury die in the motor vehicle crash that caused the brain injury. It may be a secondary effect, as friends become more distant over time or spouses file for divorce.

Persons with brain injury who are grieving require therapists to consider the effect of grieving on behavior. Typically, grieving is a process that takes time, so it is a challenge for therapists who may require more immediate behavioral change. Nonetheless, if they wish their behavioral management plan to address behavioral dyscontrol, therapists must determine the effectiveness of their plan in incorporating considerations about grieving as a phenomenological factor for a person with brain injury.

Fear

Persons with brain injury are often afraid. They may have fears based on cognitive deficits: inattention, memory, or comprehension problems which can lead to misperceptions. Misperceptions can easily trigger fear, along with anger. Alternatively, they may have fears unrelated to events and have a vague sense of insecurity and anxiety. Finally, they may be afraid of the unknown. Either their judgments about the future lead them to be afraid or the future is unfamiliar at best, and unknown at worst. When people are afraid, they fail to act rationally and are at risk for losing control.

It is crucial that therapists concentrate some of their behavioral planning on the factor of fear when it is present in persons with brain injury. Anxiety or depression can readily permeate the presentation of persons with brain injury when they are fearful. Therapists will observe withdrawal, noncompliance, and anger in response to fearfulness and related anxiety or depression.

Example: conceptualizing a phenomonology of dyscontrol

A brief example will serve to demonstrate how to conceptualize a sample phenomenology of dyscontrol. Suppose a person with brain injury presents with noncompliance to therapists' requests or directions. This person dislikes receiving assistance with activity of daily living cares. When therapists offer to help they encounter hostility, both verbal and physical. Physical aggression includes trying to strike therapists or throwing things. The person with brain injury is often late to activities because of the time necessary to complete cares. Moreover, the person voices disinterest in various activities. If the therapists push to find out what the person likes to own or enjoys participating in, they are met with denial of any interests, sarcasm, and defensiveness. When this person must interact with other persons with brain injury, there are frequent conflicts. Issues of control and domineering behavior predominate interactions.

Part of an initial evaluation and neuropsychological assessment points to the person having adequate reasoning skills but poor executive functions. Clinically, the person is willing to converse but has little trust, and attempts to end conversations whenever there is a hint of responsibility being placed on the person for the episodes of dyscontrol. In many past settings therapists have intervened to expedite care—resulting in outbursts and actually slower care completion — when executive dysfunction (now known from neuropsychological assessment) leads to disorganization and schedule disruption. Thus, previous documentation lists noncompliance with cares and aggression during cares.

After establishing rapport, therapeutic interactions eventually reveal a difficult history prior to brain injury onset. There is much dissatisfaction with relationships and significant residual bitterness. Moreover, the person believes there is little chance for a better life, particularly now with a brain injury.

Therapists gather to construct a phenomenological picture of this person from discussions with the person, neuropsychological data, and clinical observations. The person carries a lot of resentfulness from youth. This leads to a strong desire to be in control so as to avoid being hurt again, and a mistrust of others. When the therapists attempt to help with cares, they perceive their actions as evidence of their concern and good will, but the person with brain injury is leery of them, particularly of therapists who are very directive. When the therapists are directive it triggers in the person with brain injury a sense of loss of being in charge and fear about the motives of others. Hence, the person resists assistance despite the best intentions of the therapists. When the therapists respond to the person's resistance with increasing demands for compliance or by citing concerns regarding the schedule, the person with brain injury sees confirmation of the perceived low level of *real* concern the therapists have for the situation the person is in. Past utilization of rewards to motivate compliance accomplished little because of the person's disavowal of interests or enjoyment in activities. Acknowledgement of interest would reflect a willingness to let down the defensiveness that protects the person from being hurt. Finally, the alternative approach by the therapists of allowing the person to provide direction for care leads to noncompletion of the care because of executive function problems evident in the neuropsychological assessment.

As can be seen in this example, behavioral problems are determined by multiple factors that constitute the phenomenology of dyscontrol. For just this one behavior—noncompliance and its resultant aggression surrounding cares — a broad spectrum of data sources helps with phenomenological conceptualization. Therapists glean information from records, clinical observation, and trials of interaction. They note phenomenological variables including bitterness about historical factors, desire for independence, need for control, resistance to self-reflection or admission of responsibility, defensiveness, fear of being hurt, mistrust of the motives of others, a feeling of being trapped by cognitive deficits into needing help, and little hope for the future. Based on this information, therapists can devise a treatment plan that will encompass how as participants in the person's environment they might best interact with this person and how they might restructure the way in which they provide care.

Phenomenological conceptualization is complex. This example reviews an initial conceptualization of one behavior. As treatment proceeds, reconceptualization must occur as therapists gain new insights or treatment programming proves inadequate. This is just one behavior; most persons with brain injury who present with significant behavioral dyscontrol exhibit multiple behaviors for which therapists must determine the phenomenology of dyscontrol.

Conclusion

Determination of the correct phenomenology of dyscontrol is the foundation of neuropsychosocial treatment. Therapists may experience false starts in treatment when they construct an inadequate phenomenology of dyscontrol. In fact, treatment setbacks are often evidence of insufficient phenomenological conceptualization. Therapists must realize that throughout neuropsychosocial treatment, phenomenological conceptualization needs to remain fluid as they acquire greater insights about the person with behavioral dyscontrol after acquired brain injury.

References

1. Weslowski, M.D. and Zencius, A.H., *A Practical Guide to Head Injury Rehabilitation: A Focus on Posttraumatic Residential Treatment,* Plenum Press, 1994, chap. 2.
2. Treadwell, K. and Page, T.J., Functional analysis: identifying the environmental determinants of severe behavior disorders, *J. Head Trauma Rehab.,* 11, 62, 1996.
3. Karol, R.L., Rehabilitation of the injured worker from a psychological perspective, in *Industrial Therapy,* Key, G.L., Ed., Mosby, New York, 1995, chap. 18.
4. Ashley, M.J., et al., *Working with Behavior Disorders: Strategies for Traumatic Brain Injury Rehabilitation*, Psychological Corporation, San Antonio, TX, 1995, chap. 9.

chapter five

Behavior plans: application of the neuropsychosocial approach

Laura A. McDaniels

Introduction

The use of behavior plans is the key to implementing the neuropsychosocial approach in the treatment of persons with brain injury. In short, behavior plans are written descriptions of interventions used to improve a specific target behavior. Their use by therapists creates the basis for a unified team approach that results in improved behavior in persons with brain injury. The clarity and permanence of written descriptions as opposed to verbal communications, which can be misinterpreted or forgotten over time, encourages consistency across therapists. Consistent adherence to agreed-upon interventions by all therapists eliminates the confusion and frustration that persons with brain injury may experience if their therapists use conflicting approaches which, in turn, can fail to improve or even worsen behavior.

The core behavior plan is the point of departure for the creation of a behavior plan customized for a specific person with brain injury. A core behavior plan exists for each of 18 target behaviors addressed in this chapter:

1. Physical and verbal aggression
2. Poor safety/judgment
3. Risk to elope
4. Wandering
5. Somatic complaints
6. Hoarding
7. Sexually inappropriate behavior
8. Disorientation
9. Suicidal/depressive statements

10. Demanding/manipulative behavior
11. Self-injurious behavior
12. Decreased cognition
13. Hallucinations/delusions
14. Social withdrawal
15. Noncompliance
16. Unawareness of deficit
17. Socially inappropriate behavior
18. Anxiety

Core behavior plans contain the basic, most common interventions used to treat each of the above behaviors. Because of this, they can be used immediately when therapists begin to work with persons with brain injury, thus encouraging consistency of treatment from the outset. Moreover, the use of core behavior plans promotes efficiency among therapists. Rather than starting anew with each person with brain injury, creating a behavior plan from scratch by first writing down the common interventions already used for certain target behaviors, therapists can spend their time more productively by modifying these existing core behavior plans for each specific individual.

The core behavior plans that follow have been specifically developed for persons with brain injury. Although some information is applicable to other patient populations, these behavior plans were not designed to address other treatment groups. While these plans may work with other populations, the traditional treatment approaches described in Chapter 1 are also appropriate for other patient populations. The core plans do include elements of traditional approaches because it is wise to evaluate the effectiveness of these interventions early for persons with brain injury who exhibit behavioral dyscontrol as therapists build the neuropsychosocial treatment plan.

Neither the target behaviors nor the corresponding core behavior plans are meant to be exhaustive or inclusive in nature. Given the unending variations of brain injury and subsequent behavior, therapists may encounter other target behaviors. In addition, there are an almost limitless number of possible variations in the behavior plans that therapists can use to treat any given target behavior. The following core behavior plans, then, are only a starting place for therapists, who can alter them to meet the needs of individuals in treatment. Indeed, these core behavior plans will generally need additions and deletions appropriate for the unique physical, cognitive, emotional, social, and behavior deficits and abilities of specific persons with brain injury. (Chapter 8 presents examples of the types of plans that can grow from core plans.) Moreover, therapists need to customize the plans, taking into account the characteristics of the setting in which they will implement them. Persons with brain injury who therapists are called upon to treat live in many different types of settings: at home with family or in group homes, nursing facilities, or hospitals. Finally, therapists need to modify behavior plans to fit work and day program settings as well.

Behavior plans need to be both abstract and concrete in nature. They need to be abstract enough to help therapists conceptualize the problems of persons with brain injury and to provide a brief rationale for the treatment plan. The clearer the purpose of the plan at the outset, the greater the ownership of and commitment to following through with the plan therapists will have. At the same time, plans need to be concrete and very detail-oriented to facilitate consistent implementation by all therapists of the specific interventions they contain.

The availability of core behavior plans still requires therapists to attend to the phenomenology of behavioral dyscontrol. Therapists need to assess the reasons why particular behaviors occur. Attempts to implement these core plans without an accurate conceptualization of the behavior will result in failure. These plans are not a cookbook, and they do not relieve therapists from their obligation to do a thorough behavior analysis. For example, therapists should document what happens during a behavioral incident, recording what behaviors persons with brain injury display, the interventions therapists attempt, the level of success or failure of these interventions, the level of anger the persons with brain injury show and how the anger escalates, behaviors which correlate with the escalation in anger, the length of time of the behavioral incident, and how the persons eventually calm. The more that therapists know about the patterns of behavioral problems persons with brain injury experience as well as their responses to different interventions, the more effective the behavior plans will be. In brief, behavioral analysis and behavioral case conceptualization are essential with behavior plans.

Behavior plans

Physical and verbal aggression

The first behavior plan addresses the behavior that tends to cause the most distress and problems for persons with brain injury, their families, and their therapists: physical and verbal aggression. (See Table 5.1 for the core plan.) The plan for physical and verbal aggression points to the importance of assessing the external environment of persons with brain injury as well as their internal emotional state, as both elements play a role in the manifestation of aggressive behavior. Throughout the core plan for physical and verbal aggression is the neuropsychosocial focus on the therapist's actions and the environment.

First, therapists need to take into account the external environment. Persons with brain injury may become agitated by the characteristics of their physical surroundings such as the volume of noise, the number of people, or amount of activity in the room, or distractions produced by passersby. The way in which other people interact with persons with brain injury is also part of the external environment and may be of paramount importance in contributing to aggressive behavior. Second, therapists should consider the internal emotional and cognitive state of persons with brain injury who

Table 5.1 Physical and Verbal Aggression

Interventions	
1.	Label the person's emotions in an empathic manner.
2.	Label behaviors in nonjudgmental way.
3.	Redirect to activity or topic using verbal or non-verbal cues.
4.	Reapproach person at another time when possible.
5.	Distract with another activity or topic.
6.	Redirect person to a less stimulating environment.
7.	Assess for triggers of behavior (e.g., highly stimulating environment, intervention used, or person's emotional or cognitive deficits).
8.	Alter environment and treatment approach based on assessment.

engage in physical or verbal aggression. Persons with brain injury may be disoriented and may become angry when others try to reorient them. Persons with brain injury who have severe memory problems and a tendency to confabulate may become aggressive if confronted with a reality different from the one they perceive exists. Such external and internal elements will influence how therapists alter their approaches to redirect persons with brain injury to successfully prevent or reduce aggression.

After therapists have accounted for the internal and external environments, labeling the emotions of persons with brain injury by verbally stating in an empathetic manner the emotion that therapists sense is the first intervention of the core behavior plan for physical and verbal aggression. For example, a therapist may perceive that an individual with brain injury is angry and state, "You seem frustrated." Labeling emotions can help ground persons with brain injury by helping them identify and become more aware of their emotions or behaviors. This may give them an opportunity to slow down and process what they are feeling. As a result, they may be able to gain more control of their emotions and behaviors. (Therapists should note that asking what a person with brain injury is feeling without providing an observation about what the therapist perceives may at times be beneficial, but many persons with brain injury require some suggestions from which to pick. Without labels from their therapists, they may become more agitated; they may be unable to answer open-ended questions. The typical therapeutic approach of open-ended questioning before labeling may be contraindicated.)

A second intervention — labeling the behaviors of persons with brain injury — refers to verbally stating in a nonjudgmental manner what behavior therapists observe. For instance, a therapist may observe an individual change his tone of voice, swear, and threaten another person. The therapist could then state, "You are threatening that person." Because persons with brain injury who have behavior problems often have difficulty monitoring their own behavior and its appropriateness, labeling the behavior makes these persons aware of their behavior. It also allows for a feedback loop as to whether a behavior is acceptable to others.

However, labeling the feelings or behaviors of persons with brain injury may not be sufficient in helping them discontinue aggressive behavior. Therapists may need to supplement labeling with other interventions. A third intervention is verbal redirection as to how persons with brain injury should act after labeling their behavior. A case in point is that of the individual who swears and threatens others and remains agitated after the therapist labels the behavior. The therapist may state, "What is the matter? Come over here, and tell me about it," and redirect the individual to a different area. This approach helps remove persons with brain injury who are agitated from the environment that has overstimulated them by gaining their attention and shifting it to other stimuli. These persons may still be unable to calm. In such cases, the most effective intervention may be for therapists to inform them that they, the therapists, need to leave until the anger of the persons with brain injury subsides, at the same time assuring them that the therapists will return when the persons with brain injury are calm. This technique works only when therapists can ensure that the persons with brain injury will demonstrate appropriate control after the therapists leave, and only if the persons with brain injury are in a safe environment.

Reapproaching persons with brain injury who have trouble with aggressive behaviors is the fourth intervention. Persons with brain injury may become angry and aggressive when therapists attempt to do cares with them, ask them to take their medication, or invite them to go to physical or cognitive therapies. Approaching such individuals at another time when either they are calm or their environment is less stimulating may reduce or eliminate their aggression.

Distraction, the fifth intervention, is a useful strategy when persons with brain injury become aggressive. It is most appropriate with individuals who have limited attention spans. If persons with brain injury become agitated because they are unable to reach someone on the phone, for instance, therapists may distract them by talking about something happening in their immediate environment, such as eating lunch. Another distraction technique is for therapists to talk with agitated persons about something that clearly interests them personally, such as a hobby. Distraction can be even more effective if a third person can provide the distraction. As an illustration, consider the following scenario: a therapist enters the room and observes a person with brain injury yelling at another therapist. The second therapist will likely be more effective at distracting the angry individual than the first therapist, who is the target of the person's verbal aggression.

The preceding interventions may not immediately lead to a pattern of behavioral control. Aggression may persist early in treatment before therapists have fully developed a particular neuropsychosocial environment. It is useful for therapists to have access to a quiet place for persons with brain injury to retreat to when they are agitated. In rare instances, it may be necessary to have these persons escorted to the quiet place, such as their room, until they are calm. In such cases, therapists will need to modify the core plans.

Therapists commonly make several additions and deletions to the core behavior plan for aggression. As described above, primary interventions include labeling the emotions or behavior of persons with brain injury in a nonjudgmental manner. However, in some cases it may be better to avoid labeling emotions or behavior. Therapists may find through the process of refinement that some aggressive persons with brain injury may become angrier when therapists label their emotions. For example, in response to limit-setting, some persons with brain injury may clench their fists and their faces may turn red. Normally in such situations, the therapist may turn to the individual affected and state, "You look angry." This approach is often successful in helping persons recognize their emotional state and calm down. However, with some persons with brain injury, this approach may in fact escalate their anger to the point of aggression. Therapists may learn that the preferred approach for those persons is to avoid labeling emotions.

Therapists may discover that it is beneficial to delete the step of labeling the behavior and move directly to the step of redirecting persons with brain injury who are agitated to another activity or a different environment. Therapists may use phrases such as, "Let's not think about that anymore right now," or "Let's sit down and talk." In this way, they acknowledge that the persons with brain injury know that something is wrong, yet they give them an alternative activity to do. This technique can prevent the development of less desirable behaviors such as swearing or throwing things.

Persons with brain injury who have severe cognitive impairments may respond better to distraction than to either the step of labeling alone or both labeling and redirection. In such cases, distracting these persons with either something in their immediate environment or an enjoyable activity may be the desired approach. The distracting activity, however, needs to be interesting or compelling enough to successfully shift attention from the original incident. Even so, distraction is not always effective. Distraction as an intervention may need to be deleted from the behavior plans of persons with brain injury who have a good attention span. The use of redirection may be effective with them. Others may respond to distraction on some occasions and to redirection on others. Therapists need to be flexible and to read the cues given out by persons with brain injury to determine which intervention to use at any given moment.

Another common change to the behavior plan for physical and verbal aggression is to delete all three interventions mentioned above: labeling, redirection, and distraction. This is sometimes necessary in situations in which persons with brain injury lose emotional control quickly and are at risk to aggress towards themselves or others. For example, some individuals have poor awareness of their internal emotional state and do not recognize any warning signs of their growing anger. Some may not notice warning signs soon enough and, as a result, their behavior escalates. Decreasing the stimulation in these persons' environments by removing noise and/or the presence of others from their immediate surroundings to allow them to calm can be effective. Removing such individuals from the environment at hand to a quiet and safe environment may also be necessary.

Poor safety/judgment

Poor safety refers to situations in which persons with brain injury are impulsive and attempt to engage in a physical activity that places them at risk for physical harm to themselves. (See Table 5.2 for the core plan.) Most commonly, poor safety is a result of disinhibition combined with physical limitations that prohibit individuals from standing or walking independently. These persons attempt to move despite their limitations, for example, by trying to get out of bed or rising from a wheelchair on their own, when they are incapable of doing so safely.

Poor judgment refers to the lack of cognitive capacity on the part of persons with brain injury to accurately perceive, interpret, and act upon the multitude of verbal and nonverbal cues in their environment. These cues may be in the form of information about events currently taking place in their environment as well as past information from previous social or interpersonal interactions that they are unable to recall or retrieve accurately. The following incident is an example of poor judgment in action. An individual with brain injury who is socially intrusive approaches a second person with brain injury in a boisterous manner. The second person is large and physically strong, tends to be rigid and intolerant of others, and has a history of aggressing toward the first individual. The first individual does not recall being aggressed against in the past. Additionally, the first individual is unable to accurately read cues and signs or to inhibit, and therefore chooses to interact with the second person, due to poor judgment.

The first intervention in the core behavior plan for poor safety/judgment is to assess the current level of safety and judgment of the person with brain injury. Next, therapists can label or verbally identify unsafe behaviors or

***Table* 5.2** Poor Safety or Judgment

	Interventions
1.	Assess person's current level of safety and judgment and label unsafe behaviors in a nonjudgmental manner.
2.	Teach safe behaviors.
3.	Encourage use of methods to meet needs (e.g., use of call lights or verbal requests).
4.	Use environmental cues to redirect (e.g., written, pictorial, verbal, demonstration, and tactile).
5.	Create environment that minimizes risk of harm to self (e.g., keep person within eyesight, position room close to therapist, assess for use of helmet as appropriate, and remove sharp objects).
6.	Utilize rest schedules to enhance person's cognition and response to redirection.
7.	Establish walk schedule to reduce restlessness or physical discomfort.

situations of poor judgment. The labeling and identification needs to be delivered in a nonjudgmental manner to prevent agitation or escalation to aggressive behavior. The second intervention is to teach safe behaviors as the person with brain injury is able to tolerate them. The third intervention is to teach and encourage the use of call lights or other methods of receiving assistance from others. Some persons with brain injury may become agitated when therapists attempt to teach them new behaviors or procedures due to poor awareness of their physical deficits and low interest in learning. Persons with brain injury may also have such significant cognitive deficits that they cannot respond to these types of instruction and may become frustrated in response to attempts to teach them.

The fourth intervention identifies the need for therapists to provide environmental cues to redirect persons with brain injury appropriately. For example, therapists can redirect individuals who are prone to endanger themselves by rising from a wheelchair unaided by placing a written direction to stay seated on their lap tray. In the case of persons with brain injury who are aphasic, therapists can demonstrate with hand gestures the need to sit, or, alternatively, use pictures to communicate. Sometimes persons who are severely aphasic or cognitively impaired benefit from a gentle tactile cue from therapists, such as holding their hand to redirect them.

Therapists can also intervene by making adjustments in the environment of persons with brain injury to reduce the risk of injury. It may be essential to ensure that certain individuals are never left alone or out of sight to prevent them from attempting to dismantle their room or standing from their wheelchair. It may be necessary to remove any sharp or potentially harmful objects from their environment. It may also be important to separate individuals who have had a physical altercation in the past and who lack the capacity to behave differently in the present. This last intervention is particularly important for persons with poor judgment who are at risk to be harmed by others.

There are a few common deletions to the core plan for poor safety/judgment. Labeling behavior can be deleted from the plan of persons with brain injury if it agitates them. Teaching safe behaviors or how to get assistance from others can be deleted for those who lack the cognitive capacity to attend, recall, and learn new skills. These interventions may be added back into the plan at a later date if the abilities of the persons with brain injury improve to the point of these interventions becoming effective.

Risk to elope

Risk to elope is a target behavior exhibited by persons with brain injury who have talked about wanting to run away from a facility or who have actually attempted to leave a facility in the past. (See Table 5.3 for the core plan.) Therapists may also monitor this behavior when they are aware that persons with brain injury will receive news that will likely anger them and that may result in an attempt to elope.

Table 5.3 Risk to Elope

Interventions
1. Provide person with rules or guidelines of a new setting (e.g., distance from exits or level of supervision needed).
2. Utilize environmental cues to redirect from exits (e.g., different color carpet or line of tape near exits, sign on door, bell that rings when door opens, or verbal cues).
3. Distract person away from exits.
4. Reorient person if needed.
5. Discuss with person reasons for wanting to leave and provide empathy.
6. Suggest alternative solutions.
7. Identify reasons for supervised living setting, goals, and consequences of elopement based on person's cognitive abilities.
8. If person elopes, call 911.

A past history of elopement places persons with brain injury at a higher risk for future elopement. For this reason, assessment for risk to elope necessitates communication among therapists when persons with brain injury make comments about thoughts or plans to elope. It is helpful to document what events have preceded past attempts to leave or comments about a plan to leave. Discussing the reasons for persons with brain injury wanting to leave and then helping them meet their needs can reduce their desire to leave and help calm them down if they are angry or aroused. Empathizing with such persons and paraphrasing their feelings can help them feel understood and may result in their relaxing and deciding to stay. Suggesting alternative solutions to their problems can be useful if they show poor problem solving abilities.

Persons with brain injury are often unaware of the reasons they may need to be in a supervised setting. They may lack insight into the problems they have that require assistance from others. Discussing these reasons can improve their understanding and acceptance of their current setting. Some persons with brain injury have difficulty handling the consequences of their behavior. They may respond to emotional stress in an impulsive manner by attempting to run away from their setting or, in essence, from their problems. Therapists need to intervene with persons with brain injury who have such difficulties by encouraging them to take extra time to think rather than acting immediately. Identifying potential consequences for running away in a calm and non-threatening manner can also assist persons with brain injury in making better choices.

Providing persons with brain injury with the rules or guidelines of the setting where they live or work at the time they begin there can prevent some future misunderstandings. For example, some facilities such as hospitals may have rules about how close persons with brain injury can be to the exits. In other cases, cueing them to existing physical markers such as the presence of a different color of carpet near exits reduces risk of elopement and gives persons with cognitive impairment concrete cues to follow.

Sometimes, persons with brain injury who are disoriented may walk to a door and push on it. They may simply turn around after a minute or so if the door is locked, and they are unsuccessful in leaving. In this situation, direct intervention from therapists is unnecessary. However, therapists may want to distract these persons with another activity after they walk away from the door.

Therapists can delete the intervention of suggesting alternative solutions to the problems of persons with brain injury from this core behavior plan if such persons are disoriented and at risk for elopement. In such cases, it would be more practical to attempt to orient them to place and situation. In contrast, when persons with brain injury who are oriented decide that they want to leave a facility, the plan should emphasize finding alternative solutions to their problems. Therapists might encourage them to speak with their family, legal decision maker, case manager, physician, or group home coordinator about moving to another facility instead of eloping.

Wandering

Persons with brain injury who show poor ability to find their way around the facility in which they reside manifest wandering behavior. (See Table 5.4 for the core plan.) Wandering behavior is due to cognitive impairments and often occurs when persons with brain injury are in a new, unfamiliar setting. The behavior generally improves over time as the persons become familiar with the setting.

The first intervention of the core behavior plan for wandering is to monitor for safety. There are times when individuals may wander into the rooms of others and may be at risk for the persons with brain injury living in those rooms to aggress against them. When persons first arrive at a new setting, therapists should explain to them in simple, concrete terms the need to stay in an assigned area. The key to implementing this plan is for therapists to observe persons with brain injury as closely as possible, particularly when they exhibit wandering behavior.

Table 5.4 Wandering

Interventions
1. Monitor for safety.
2. Explain to the person the need to stay in assigned area. Use simple concrete terms.
3. Mark the environment (e.g., write name or place picture on bedroom door; use different colors of carpet or a line of tape on floor; place signs for person to turn around or stop at exits).
4. Assess reasons for wandering and attempt to meet needs.
5. Reorient as needed.
6. Attempt distraction.
7. Label and redirect when person is leaving assigned area.

Marking the environment can be extremely effective in reducing wandering behavior. The most common visual cue to help persons with brain injury is to place their name on the door of their room. Putting a colorful, attention-getting picture on the door is an effective alternative for persons who have trouble reading. Sometimes a photograph of the person with brain injury on his or her door is a valuable intervention. In addition, a change in the look of the physical environment from one area to another assists them in knowing in which area they need to stay. For example, the use of a variety of colors of carpet to differentiate the areas that persons with brain injury need to stay within from prohibited areas (such as therapist areas and exits) can be extremely effective. Placing tape on the floor can accomplish the same goal if larger physical plant changes cannot be made. Similarly, a large sign hung at eye level can successfully redirect persons from wandering out of an area, especially if names are used on the sign to attract the attention of individuals at risk for wandering.

Other techniques may also be appropriate in treating persons with brain injury who wander. Assessing the reason for wandering can at times reduce the behavior. For example, if therapists learn that persons with brain injury who wander often mistakenly go into someone else's room as they look for their own, they can help these individuals find their own room. Another strategy that therapists can use when finding persons in someone else's room is to ask them if the personal items in the room look familiar to them. They may be more receptive to redirection away from the room if they do not recognize any items. The repetition of interventions when persons attempt to leave assigned areas often results in reduced wandering behavior over time.

Somatic complaints

Therapists label preoccupation with physical sensations or discomfort as somatic complaints. This preoccupation makes it difficult for persons with brain injury to engage in meaningful activities. (See Table 5.5 for the core plan.) Often there may be a physical basis for the complaints, though the magnitude of the complaints may be exaggerated. Sometimes the complaints have more of a psychological than medical etiology. In either case, in the neuropsychosocial approach, therapists' responses to the somatic complaints are crucial.

Obviously, somatic complaints should be evaluated to determine any underlying organic pathology. Appropriate treatment should commence if medical caregivers find a treatable physical condition. Therapists should avoid succumbing to the temptation to assume that somatic complaints are illegitimate among persons with brain injury just because persons with brain injury fail to articulate their symptoms as well as others might. It is equally important for therapists to keep persons with brain injury up to date on the results of their tests and evaluations and informed about their progress in treatment to further enhance behavioral control. Frustration about being kept

***Table* 5.5** Somatic Complaints

Interventions
1. Evaluate and treat all medical problems.
2. Provide person with feedback on test results and progress.
3. Assess situational stressors and triggers of somatic complaints.
4. Reassure person and acknowledge concerns and fears.
5. Encourage person to express feelings and listen in nonjudgmental manner.
6. Initiate coping skills based on cognitive abilities: for example, suggest taking a few deep breaths (relaxation techniques) or offer possible solutions (problem solving techniques).
7. Normalize new physical sensations.
8. Provide social attention for appropriate behaviors.
9. Redirect or distract to another topic or activity.

in the dark about their condition can lead persons with brain injury to behavioral dyscontrol. Of course, therapists should present such information in a fashion that persons with brain injury can understand given their particular cognitive deficits.

Sometimes situational stressors accompany somatic complaints, and the stressors trigger the symptoms. Such stressors may be present when the complaints are primarily organic or when they are mostly psychological. Therapists should continue to examine the nature and pattern of somatic complaints for neuropsychosocial variables even when there is a clear physical aspect to the complaint. For example, a person with brain injury presents with stomach distress and vomiting that leads to missing therapy. Therapists determine that there has been poor progress in therapy. The emotional turmoil from failure in therapy causes physical illness. Therapists who attend to the underlying issue of poor coping with treatment struggles can ameliorate the health condition.

Reassurance about physical problems and possible underlying stressors can assist persons with brain injury in their coping. It is also important for therapists to help persons with brain injury to express their feelings about both their overall situation and their physical symptoms. Many persons with brain injury may otherwise feel uncomfortable directly relating their emotional status. When they are able to disclose their feelings about their general status there is less likelihood that stress will lead to physical symptoms, because they will feel less stressed. When they relate their feelings about physical symptoms they will also cope better, because such disclosure tends to provide a sense of not being alone with health problems. Sharing emotions with other people helps relieve stress.

It is often necessary to use an indirect approach to increase the sense of safety that persons with brain injury who display somatic complaints may require to disclose their feelings. An environment that encourages relaxation, perhaps even supplemented with relaxation training or other responses when angry (e.g., problem solving) can help with coping, but therapists must very carefully consider cognitive deficits when complementing the neuropsychosocial approach with skill building.

Sometimes persons with brain injury are hypervigilant about their physical condition. They may be oversensitive to changes in physical condition and to sensory input from their bodies. Their response may be more dramatic than therapists might expect. Also, they may be anxious or angry about their condition, which exacerbates their responses. The neuropsychosocial approach outlined in other sections can address the subsequent aggression, noncompliance, etc. that comprise their excessive responses. Sometimes therapists can also assist them by normalizing the new sensations.

A common response to physical changes that deserves special mention is attention-seeking behavior. Persons with brain injury may receive most of their attention, social interaction, and emotional support when they complain about physical symptoms. This may lead to unintentional exaggeration of these symptoms to ensure ongoing attention. Therapists can create a neuropsychosocial world in which social attention is available in other ways than in regard to physical symptoms. An enriched environment is conducive to broader interests and can distract from physical status.

Hoarding

Hoarding behavior refers to the gathering and storing of excessive amounts of objects or food. (See Table 5.6 for the core plan.) This behavior can manifest itself in a variety of ways and may have undesirable consequences. For example, some persons with brain injury collect certain types of food with the intention of storing them. When they store perishable items at room temperature, a health problem results when the food begins to decompose. Persons with brain injury can also hoard objects ranging from large items such as exercise equipment to small, seemingly irrelevant items such as packages of salt and pepper. Hoarding objects often first becomes a problem

Table 5.6 Hoarding

Interventions
1. Monitor for hoarding of food or property.
2. Observe for stealing of others food or property.
3. Identify antecedents of hoarding behavior.
4. Assess for underlying cause of the behavior (e.g., anxiety, need to control, disinhibition or impulsivity).
5. Reduce stressors in environment and allow person to have control over their own objects as much as possible to reduce hoarding.
6. Teach self-control techniques to reduce disinhibition and impulsivity based on cognitive abilities.
7. If person steals food, alter environment so that person eats alone or at safe distance from others.
8. Set reasonable limits on the number of items the person can have access to.
9. Routinely check living space and remove excess items.

when persons with brain injury become so preoccupied with hoarding rituals that they are unable to fully participate in more productive activities. Hoarding can become such a problem that the amount of items collected becomes so excessive that there is no room left in the individuals' living space to accommodate the items. The living space may become so cluttered that there is no longer enough space to complete cares. Individuals who hoard large numbers of objects tend to lose their items easily. Furthermore, excessive clutter can become a fire hazard.

Hoarding is sometimes accomplished by stealing. Some persons with brain injury steal food from others with the intent to save and store it. Some steal objects as well as food. Stealing food or objects can create interpersonal problems with roommates or other residents. Roommates may become aggressive toward people who steal from them. In addition, sometimes there are legal consequences for stealing.

The first two interventions of the core behavior plan for hoarding are to monitor and to observe persons for hoarding and stealing behaviors. Persons with brain injury can often be secretive about hoarding or stealing if they are aware that such behaviors are unusual or unacceptable to others. Thus, therapists need to stay alert to hoarding behavior in order to prevent it from escalating. Labeling and redirecting the attention of persons who hoard may work if the behavior is not severe or ingrained. Providing these persons with feedback about how their behavior is disruptive to others or is unsafe may be helpful for persons with cognitive strengths in reasoning and memory, and fairly good self-control. When the above approaches are ineffective, therapists need to focus treatment on changing the environment to reduce hoarding behavior.

The third intervention is to identify the antecedents of the hoarding behavior. This strategy facilitates the next intervention — assessing the underlying cause of the behavior — and provides insight into additional interventions. For example, if an individual who hoards show signs of anxiety before a visitor arrives and repeatedly steals from the visitor or hoards objects before or after the visit, anxiety about the visit, the visitor, or the topics to be discussed during the visit may be the cause of the behavior. Persons who suffer from anxiety may compulsively hoard in an attempt to reduce anxiety. For these persons, identifying and attempting to reduce the stressors in their environment can reduce their level of anxiety, which ultimately reduces their compulsive hoarding behavior. Another reason persons hoard objects is to give themselves a sense of security by having control over something. In such cases, helping persons have control over objects of their own or over events can reduce their need to hoard.

Other causes of hoarding behavior are disinhibition and impulsivity. Persons with brain injury may have deficits in their ability to judge at a given moment what behavior is acceptable, or to stop and think before acting. For instance, the impulsive individual who lives in a group setting and tends to hoard food sees a brownie on another person's plate at lunchtime. Without thinking, the first individual lunges for the brownie. Strategies exist to treat hoarding behavior that results from impulsivity and disinhibition problems. Therapists may start by teaching self-control techniques so that persons with brain injury relearn the ability to stop and think before acting. Some individuals are able to benefit from learning which situations they tend to act impulsively in, and to prepare ahead of time for how they plan to act in those situations. Another technique that these persons can learn is to say the word "stop" out loud or to themselves, or to simply walk away from situations to prevent impulsive responses.

Although therapists may attempt to teach such self-control techniques, the techniques often prove to be ineffective. In these cases, therapists must use neuropsychosocial strategies. For example, therapists may have persons who steal food from others at mealtimes — and, as a result, are at risk to be aggressed against — either eat alone or at a safe distance from others. They may also set reasonable limits on the number of items to which persons with brain injury can have access, in order to prevent hoarding of objects. Therapists may need to routinely check the living spaces, clothes, notebooks, etc. of persons with brain injury who hoard, and remove excess items.

Sexually inappropriate behavior

Sexually inappropriate behavior refers to sexual behavior that is socially unacceptable or without mutual consent. (See Table 5.7 for the core plan.) The behavior can be explicit, such as when a person grabs another's breasts, groin, or buttock area, or it can be less blatant but still clearly sexual, such as touching another person's leg, attempting to kiss or rub into someone in a sexual manner, or touching any part of another's body in a sexual manner.

Table 5.7 Sexually Inappropriate Behavior

	Interventions
1.	Label sexually inappropriate behavior and direct person to discontinue behavior (e.g., "You are touching me. Do not touch me.")
2.	Provide feedback as to how this behavior impacts others (e.g., "I feel uncomfortable when you touch me.")
3.	Distract or redirect to another topic or activity.
4.	Remove individual from setting or from person whom they are targeting sexually.
5.	Leave and reapproach when person is calm.
6.	Use only male or female therapists based on person's behavior.
7.	Offer opportunities to express emotions and socialize in an appropriate manner.
8.	Utilize sensory stimulation as needed.
9.	Redirect to use alternative socially acceptable behaviors (e.g., shake hands rather than grabbing others).
10.	Respond to attention seeking behavior with flat affect and matter-of-fact tone of voice.
11.	Set limits and boundaries by clarifying roles.

Requests for sex, sexual comments, or sexual jokes are less dramatic examples, yet they can be quite offensive to others. Other offensive behaviors include masturbating in public, disrobing or exposing oneself to others, getting into another resident's bed without clothes on, inserting objects into the vagina or anus, asking therapists to help with bathroom cares that individuals are capable of doing themselves, and standing too close to others in a suggestive fashion.

The first interventions of the core behavior plan for sexually inappropriate behavior are to label the behavior and direct the persons with brain injury to discontinue the behavior. For example, if an individual reaches out and attempts to touch a therapist's breast, the therapist can say, "You tried to touch me sexually, and I do not like that. Do not touch me." In such cases, it is important that therapists remain calm so that the persons with brain injury acting inappropriately can calm down and process cognitively what they are saying. Other interventions focus on processing and reasoning with the persons with brain injury as to why the behavior is unacceptable. This is helpful if the persons with brain injury believe that the behavior is acceptable and have the cognitive abilities to reason and recall information. Therapists should delete these interventions when the persons with brain injury lack the memory, reasoning, or impulse control abilities to prevent future behaviors. Another intervention is to distract or redirect persons who behave in a sexually inappropriate manner to another activity or topic. Removing them from a particular area or moving them away from the person toward whom they are behaving inappropriately is generally useful. Therapists can also remove themselves from the situation and return when the individual exhibiting sexually inappropriate behavior is calm.

It is crucial that therapists implement the neuropsychosocial approach in such cases in addition to emphasizing skill building. Altering the neuropsychosocial environment can almost always be effective. For instance, one intervention, when feasible, is to have only male therapists assist persons who are sexually inappropriate exclusively with female therapists. This, of course, is appropriate also for the reverse scenario: assigning only female therapists to persons who are inappropriate with male therapists. It may be necessary to separate certain persons during daily activities or change their room assignments if one individual targets another sexually.

Persons with brain injury may display sexually inappropriate behavior for reasons that are not easily apparent. Some may show severe cognitive impairments or language problems, and thus fail at attempts to connect with others in a socially acceptable fashion. This can lead to feelings of loneliness and social isolation. Offering these persons opportunities to express their thoughts and feelings through talking, nonverbal communication, or socializing in a group can reduce their inappropriate behaviors. Other persons with brain injury may lack sensory stimulation and not receive much human touch except during cares. As a result, they may grab their therapists sexually during cares. Therapists can attempt sensory stimulation programs that may help them decrease such behaviors. They can direct persons with brain injury who are very concrete and perseverate on sexual behaviors, such as grabbing at others, to place their hand on the arm of their chair (repeatedly, if necessary). They can give persons who try to hug or grab them socially acceptable alternative behaviors to use to meet their needs. For example, therapists can set limits with such persons by stating that they can shake hands instead. Therapists must take care to ensure that persons with brain injury do not try the alternatives they institute continually. Limiting shaking hands to the beginning and the end of an interaction may be necessary if persons with brain injury attempt to shake hands constantly.

Therapists can create an environment in which they adopt a flat affect, avoiding a display of emotion — whether it is disgust or laughter — and use a matter-of-fact tone of voice with redirection to assist in decreasing these types of behavior. This approach applies to many attention-seeking behaviors such as masturbating, disrobing, or exposing oneself in public. The goal in such cases is not just to end the current behavior, but also to decrease the likelihood of it reoccurring. When displays of sexually inappropriate behavior occur in front of a group, removing the audience for whom the persons with brain injury are performing is essential. Therapists must remember to provide praise and much social attention for appropriate behavior, while responding in a neutral manner to inappropriate sexual behavior.

When persons with brain injury make sexual comments to therapists, therapists can lead them to a discussion in which they can explore their feelings about the limitations their injury imposes upon them. These discussions can be an opportunity for therapists to set limits and demonstrate that sexual comments lead to a review of boundaries issues and brain injury, rather than the intimate discussion they might have hoped would occur. Although this type of intervention is again most appropriate with persons who have strong cognitive strengths, boundary and limit setting can be helpful for most persons with brain injury who exhibit sexually inappropriate behavior. For persons with brain injury who have severe cognitive deficits, the limits need to be concrete and simple. It is important for therapists to be direct about what behaviors are unacceptable and to avoid couching descriptions in terms that might be misunderstood.

Limit setting typically entails therapists setting boundaries by clarifying their role and the nature of their relationship with persons with brain injury. They can identify the types of relationships that persons with brain injury can have with others, and discuss appropriate persons with whom to have personal friendships or sexual relationships. Problem solving as to how and where to meet someone with whom to have a personal relationship can also be helpful.

Disorientation

Therapists apply the term disorientation when persons with brain injury do not know the date, their location, or personal information about themselves. They may also not understand their current situation accurately. For

Table 5.8 Disorientation

Interventions
1. Assess and document patterns of fluctuating orientation (e.g., a person is more disoriented and agitated in the afternoon).
2. Establish a rest schedule.
3. Reorient person as needed.
4. Use indirect approach if orientation agitates person (e.g., "It is snowing outside.")
5. Utilize written or pictorial cues to reorient person (e.g., name or picture on bedroom door, photographs of person with family or friends, calendar, clock, and memory notebook with orientation section).
6. Reduce environmental stimulation.
7. Provide consistent therapists.

example, they may think they are part of the hospital staff. (See Table 5.8 for the core plan.) Persons with brain injury may be disoriented to one or all of the above. Persons with brain injury may engage in behaviors that are problematic due to their disorientation, such as an agitated type of aggression, wandering or inadvertent elopement, or unsafe behaviors. They may think that they are at work when they are actually in the hospital. They may decide to leave and, when therapists intervene, may then become agitated and strike out.

When orientation is variable, it is helpful to monitor and document at what time of day disorientation occurs and for how long persons with brain injury remain disoriented. This information is useful because they may be better oriented and their mood may be calmer at certain times of the day. For example, they may be poorly oriented and more agitated in the afternoon. Afternoon disorientation may be due to fatigue. Establishing a rest schedule can help prevent these problems at times.

It important for therapists to know the emotional state of persons with brain injury when they are disoriented (e.g., calm or agitated) and their response to reorientation. Some persons with brain injury can become angry and show an increase in agitation when therapists reorient them. In these circumstances, avoiding direct orientation and using a more indirect approach can assist in reorientation. For instance, a therapist can reorient an individual to the season and date by saying, "It is getting cold outside. It is almost winter. I am looking forward to Thanksgiving next week."

Written or pictorial cues are also helpful in reorienting persons with brain injury. These cues may be less threatening or embarrassing for some people than verbal orientation. They may be more consistent and practical as well. For example, it is not always possible in some settings to verbally reorient persons every time they try to find their room. Instead, therapists can place a name or picture on the door, appropriate for the persons' abilities, to reorient them. For persons who are aphasic, pictures may be effective.

Suicidal/depressive statements

Suicidal statements are verbal indications that persons with brain injury plan to kill themselves. Depressive statements are a verbal expression of their feelings of subjective sadness. (See Table 5.9 for the core plan.) When persons with brain injury make suicidal statements or show behaviors that suggest to others that they are considering suicide, therapists must take immediate steps to keep them safe.

Once persons with brain injury have made suicidal statements, therapists should assess them for suicidal thoughts, statements, plans to harm themselves, preferred method, intent to act, immediacy of intent, and access to weapons or potential objects that could be used to harm themselves. Therapists should also assess for any previous history of suicide ideation, threats, or attempts. They should determine any recent stressful events, any recent unusual behavior, and any family history of suicide. Any reasons that would prevent them from acting out a suicide such as faith, family obligations, or fear should be explored. Therapists also need to inform the rest of the team and solicit their help in suicide prevention.

Engaging persons with brain injury in coping strategies such as problem solving, socialization, expression of feelings, and relaxation skills can assist them in dealing with their strong emotions. Therapists should praise them for verbalizing their feelings and thoughts of suicide and encourage them to continue to tell others when they feel suicidal or depressed so that they

Table 5.9 Suicidal/Depressive Statements

	Interventions
1.	Following suicidal statements assess for suicidal thoughts, statements, plans, preferred method, intent to act, immediacy of intent, and access to weapons/method.
2.	Determine recent stressful events, recent unusual behavior, history of past ideation/attempts/threats, family history of suicide, and reasons that would prevent acting out suicide.
3.	Inform team and solicit help in suicide prevention.
4.	Engage person in coping strategies (e.g., problem solving, socialization, expression of feelings, and relaxation skills).
5.	Identify concrete plan with person as to whom to talk with when experiencing suicidal thoughts.
6.	Remove from environment any means person has to harm self (e.g., cords, call lights, belts, shoelaces, razors, knives, and other sharp objects).
7.	Therapist should dispense all medications to person to prevent medication overdose, if person made suicidal statements.
8.	If person needs crisis hospitalization, provide face-to-face supervision while awaiting transfer.
9.	Call 911 if need emergency assistance.
10.	Address chronic ideation with emotionally supportive environment that also facilitates problem solving.

can receive assistance. It can be useful to have them identify specific persons with whom they can talk to at these times and have a concrete plan in place at all times delineating how to respond to suicidal behavior.

Procedures for managing suicidal ideation or behaviors on behavioral hospital units are often well standardized. It is important to provide a safe and secure environment. At minimum, it is essential to remove any means that persons with brain injury have to harm themselves. It is particularly important to eliminate any means or method that they may have indicated to be part of a plan or that they have used in the past. For example, if they state that they have thought about strangling themselves with the cord of their call light, therapists should immediately remove the light and all cords and devices that could be used to strangle oneself from the living space. Common personal items to remove from the environment of persons with brain injury on suicidal precaution status in a hospital include, in addition to cords or call lights, belts, shoelaces, and any sharp objects. Most behavior units do not allow razors or knives. Therapists should remove these items from persons with brain injury if the unit otherwise allowed them to have them. In addition, therapists should dispense all medications to persons with brain injury who have made suicidal statements if they normally take their own, to prevent storing of medications and overdosing. Finally, therapists need to know the policies and procedures of their facility as well as state regulations and reporting laws as related to this type of high-risk behavior.

Managing suicidal behavior can be particularly difficult for persons with brain injury who live in community-based settings. Therapists need to consider transferring them to a crisis program for persons with brain injury or, if such a crisis program is not available, to a hospital psychiatric crisis unit for stabilization. While awaiting this transfer, it is important to provide these persons with one-to-one supervision (face to face) in a safe and secure environment. Precautions similar to those of a hospital unit should be taken. As an emergency backup, but still while providing face-to-face supervision, therapists in community settings can call 911 to get help.

In the long run, environmental changes can help address chronic suicidal or depressive ideation. An environment that provides ongoing emotional support and problem solving assistance can facilitate avoidance of depression and suicidal thoughts. Therapists can structure the neuropsychosocial environment so that it presents only challenges with which the person with brain injury can adequately cope.

Demanding/manipulative behavior

Excessive or constant requests of others in an impolite or irritable manner is called demanding behavior. Manipulative behavior can at times accompany demanding behavior, but they do not always occur together. Manipulate behavior is defined as the use of others in a negative way to achieve an end, and can involve altering the truth or outright lying. This behavior often

Table 5.10 Demanding/Manipulative Behavior

	Interventions
1.	Speak to person in a quiet, one-on-one setting when addressing behavior.
2.	Encourage person to express concerns and feelings.
3.	Offer concrete plan of action or solution.
4.	Focus person's attention on own behavior rather than demands.
5.	Assign a primary therapist and direct all requests to primary therapist.
6.	Redirect to topic or activity.
7.	Utilize a request sheet.
8.	When manipulative, provide choices to increase person's sense of control.
9.	Avoid power struggles by: being flexible, setting limits on important issues, and providing a brief rationale for limits.
10.	Be consistent in limit setting and overall plan.

comes in the form of attempting to pit therapists against one another. (See Table 5.10 for the core plan.)

Interventions one through five in the core behavior plan for demanding/manipulative behavior apply to both types of behaviors. Consistent with the neuropsychosocial approach, it is best to speak to persons with brain injury in a quiet, one-on-one situation rather than in a public setting when addressing their demands or managing their manipulative behavior. It is important to remain objective and professional. Because these behaviors can trigger frustration and defensiveness in therapists, they may be tempted to respond to this type of behavior by raising their voices, becoming short-tempered, being sarcastic, or ignoring the persons with brain injury. These types of emotional responses by therapists will likely lead to an escalation of behavior problems. In such cases, it is important for therapists to pause and prepare their thoughts prior to an encounter by reviewing their strategies and goals for the session. Therapists can respond effectively to manipulative behavior by conceptualizing persons with brain injury as attempting to gain control over their situations through means that are ineffective rather than viewing them as having personality disorders. This former conceptualization is more collaborative and less judgmental, and thus helps therapists improve the behavior of persons with brain injury.

Creating an environment in which therapists encourage persons with brain injury to express their feelings can help them focus more on their real concerns and less on their demands. The more effectively persons with brain injury can identify their needs and emotions, the easier it is to help them address these needs. As a result, it is likely that they will then make less excessive demands. When possible, providing them with concrete plans of action or solutions to meet their requests can reduce their demanding behavior as well. Consistent follow-through on plans to meet their needs or requests is essential in maintaining their trust.

Redirecting the attention of persons with brain injury to their own behavior in response to demands can also reduce the demands. For example, an individual may state, "The therapists won't get me a soda." The therapist may respond, "Why do you think they won't get you a soda?" The therapist can then explain that the reason therapists do not respond immediately to get a soda is because of this person making this request every ten minutes. If the individual lacks insight into the impact of excessive requests and the resulting lack of response by therapists, then suggestions about why this occurs can be helpful. This approach can be used for manipulative behavior as well. In either case, it is important to assign a primary therapist to them. The assigned therapist should handle all requests by a particular person with brain injury. Other therapists should direct persons with brain injury to their primary therapist when they act demanding or manipulative. This intervention alone can reduce behaviors significantly if followed consistently, because it produces an environment that prevents persons with brain injury from therapist splitting.

Additional interventions focus primarily on the reduction of demanding behaviors. Persons with brain injury who have attentional problems may interrupt an activity by making a demand. They will likely respond to a cue to refocus on the activity. This redirection also sends the message that the activity is important and that interruptions are unacceptable if persons with brain injury appear to be intentionally attempting to disrupt an activity.

The use of a request sheet can be a useful technique in managing excessive requests or demands. Request sheets are an environmental tool that allow persons with brain injury to write down and keep track of all their requests so that therapists can review them periodically, typically on an hourly basis or within a time frame based on the abilities, behaviors, and needs of the person with a brain injury. Persons with brain injury usually accept and appreciate this technique, as it assures them that their therapists will hear and address their needs. However, it is important to monitor the amount of time devoted to reviewing and attempting to meet requests, especially if the process is so time-consuming that the intervals between reviews of request sheets becomes very short. Therapists can remedy this problem by lengthening intervals between requests and negotiating adjustments in the time frame with the persons with brain injury.

An intervention that is generally effective in working with persons with brain injury who act manipulative is to provide them with choices. Lack of control over their situation can lead persons with brain injury to manipulative behavior as they attempt to gain control over what seem to be insignificant issues. This can result in a power struggle if therapists are unaware of this dynamic. Providing choices to persons with brain injury, in contrast, helps them have a greater sense of control over their situation. Choices, however, have to be acceptable for therapists as well as for the persons with brain injury. It is usually best for therapists to remain flexible and allow persons with brain injury to make decisions and do activities within their abilities as long as they are not at risk to harm themselves or others. Therapists, though, will likely still need to set limits on important issues or situations, and they should set them in a respectful yet firm manner. Providing a brief rationale for limits when persons with brain injury are able to benefit from it will also give them a greater sense of control and respect. Finally, limits need to be consistent. Consistency of the limits and of the entire behavior plan is the cornerstone of reducing manipulative behaviors.

Self-injurious behavior

Self-injurious behavior refers to when persons with brain injury engage in an act that is physically harmful to them. (See Table 5.11 for the core plan.) The behavior may take the form of them cutting themselves, swallowing sharp objects or toxic substances, biting or scratching themselves, banging their head repeatedly, or banging part of their body against a wall, bed, or other object. This behavior may be related to a depressed or angry mood. It may also result from severe cognitive, language, or physical deficits. It need not reflect a personality disorder. It may include them trying to take their life, though not necessarily.

The initial approach that therapists can use during a crisis situation is to redirect or distract persons with brain injury when they engage in self-injurious behavior. If this is ineffective, therapists should remove any objects from the environment that they are using to inflict harm on themselves. Therapists will need to physically intervene as necessary to protect them from harm. Therapists may also need to arrange for medical care if persons with brain injury have inflicted harm on themselves. If they are in the community and cannot stop the behavior or continue to be at risk for harm to self, then therapists need to arrange for crisis hospitalization.

Consistent with the neuropsychosocial approach, therapists need to make changes to the physical environment of persons with brain injury after they exhibit self-injurious behavior or when they are at risk for this behavior. These changes involve removing any objects persons have used in the past to inflict self-harm as well as preventing access to any potentially harmful

Table 5.11 Self-Injurious Behavior

Interventions
1. Redirect or distract person when engaging in behaviors.
2. If ineffective, physically intervene by removing objects person is using to inflict harm to self.
3. Arrange for medical care if person inflicted harm to self.
4. If person cannot stop behavior or is at ongoing risk of harm to self, arrange for crisis hospitalization.
5. Remove objects person has used in past to harm self and potentially harmful objects (e.g., knives, utensils, razors, scissors, long cords, matches, lighters, or cigarettes).
6. Assess need to dispense all medications to prevent overdose.
7. Assess level of supervision needed (e.g., one on one or monitoring every 15 minutes).
8. Assess underlying causes of behavior and treat accordingly.

objects or substances, including sharp objects such as knives, utensils, razors, scissors, and tools; long cords, such as those that are part of some call lights or drapes, that can be used for strangulation; and matches, lighters, or cigarettes. Therapists may also need to dispense all medications themselves if there is any risk of hoarding medication by persons with brain injury and, consequently, a potential for overdose. Therapists must be sure the persons with brain injury swallow the medications. The therapists also need to determine what type of supervision is required to maintain safety. One-on-one supervision or monitoring every fifteen minutes may be necessary for persons who exhibit self-injurious behavior, even in a seemingly safe environment.

Therapists can create an environment that supports alternatives to self-injurious behavior. They can encourage these persons to express their feelings verbally rather than acting out their emotions in harmful ways. Alternatively, therapists can shift the attention of persons with brain injury to focus on their thinking rather than on their emotions, particularly in the case of persons with brain injury who have poor emotional control. For example, in the case of persons with brain injury who are catastrophizing their situation, therapists may ask them to recall what they do to calm themselves down. Reassurance and reminders of previous successes in gaining self-control are often encouraging. Persons with poor self-esteem will benefit if therapists identify their strengths — this alone can reduce self-injurious behavior.

Some persons with brain injury will find an environment that facilitates more physical means to release emotional tension helpful. Opportunities to walk and exercise may help. An environment that provides a private area to yell or cry for a brief period of time will assist some persons with brain injury to avoid self injurious behavior. Others may find creative outlets to release emotional energy through art, music, poetry, or journaling.

Persons with brain injury may engage in self-injurious behavior in a manipulative manner. They may be angry that they are unable to get their way about something or that therapists have set a limit. They may feel out of control, rejected, or abandoned. As a result, they may respond to these feelings by engaging in self-injurious behavior. Therapists need to respond in turn by being supportive while still setting and maintaining stable boundaries and limits. Consistent staffing or, at minimum, excellent communication among therapists regarding appropriate approaches with persons with brain injury is essential to setting and maintaining boundaries.

Some persons with brain injury may show perseverative self-injurious behaviors such as biting or banging their wheelchair repeatedly into the wall. This may occur for a number of reasons. First, there may be a need for increased sensory stimulation. For instance, they may bite themselves repeatedly to obtain increased stimulation. In such cases, they may benefit from having occupational therapists initially provide sensory integration therapy. If useful, this can become part of their neuropsychosocial environment by having other therapists provide this routinely. Second, severe language and cognitive deficits may lead to perseverative behavior. Persons with brain injury who bang their wheelchair into the wall may be attempting to communicate with others. They may be trying to get a need met because they are hungry or want to use the bathroom. If therapists attempt to anticipate and address their physical needs it may help in decreasing this behavior. Sometimes persons with brain injury who are unable to speak may engage in these types of behaviors to get social attention from others. Therapists can help by identifying the most effective communication strategies to use with them (e.g., using simple yes/no questions, consistent non-verbal gestures for yes and no, communicating with an augmentative device, or using a letter or picture board). These methods become part of the world of persons with brain injury.

Decreased cognition

Decreased cognition, within the context of a behavior plan, refers to cognitive problems that are so prominent in the conceptualization of behavioral problems that a plan to address these issues has a positive impact on other behaviors and overall functioning. (See Table 5.12 for the core plan.) The cognitive difficulties may be global or specific in nature, such as impairments in attention, memory, language, perception, perseveration, initiation, or problem solving.

The first intervention for decreased cognition is to keep the environment simple and free from clutter. A cluttered and over-stimulating environment can increase emotional arousal level, leading, in turn, to behavior problems. In contrast, a simple, low-stimulation environment helps maximize the application of the functional capacity of persons with brain injury.

It is also helpful for persons with brain injury to have adequate rest. The likelihood of persons with brain injury displaying a behavior problem tends to be higher when they are tired, because they demonstrate a lowered cognitive ability to control behavior when they are tired. Therefore, encouraging them to have adequate rest can reduce behavior difficulties.

Table 5.12 Decreased Cognition

Interventions
1. Keep environment simple, free from clutter, and quiet.
2. Encourage adequate rest.
3. Provide structure with written daily routine and keep changes to a minimum.
4. Make eye contact before speaking.
5. Use one on one interventions when possible or speak to person one at a time.
6. Keep interactions brief and use concrete one step requests.
7. Provide repetition and allow person extra time to process information.
8. Utilize written, pictorial, verbal, and tactile cues (e.g., memory notebook, name or picture on bedroom door, calendar, clock and watch).
9. Present small amounts of material in an organized manner.

Providing structure for persons with brain injury is extremely important in enhancing their functioning. As it can be difficult for them to internally organize their thinking and control their emotions following brain injury, a structured lifestyle can reduce stress and help them succeed. A written daily routine provides a framework for achieving needed structure. Within this framework, any changes in the living, work, leisure, or day program setting should be kept to a minimum due to the high cognitive demands of adjusting and adapting to new environments, people, and routines. In addition, consistency in staffing should be paramount, as persons with brain injury may have problems adjusting to the subtleties of style and personalities of new therapists.

Several strategies can be used with persons with cognitive deficits to facilitate their understanding and recall, and thus improve their behavior. First, it is often helpful to make eye contact before speaking to them, to gain their attention. This is also necessary when initiating communication with persons with brain injury who are non-verbal. Second, one-on-one interactions are generally easier for persons with brain injury to process than group interactions. When one-to-one communication is not possible, it is best to have therapists talk one at a time to assist the persons with brain injury in attending and tracking the conversation. On the other hand, if they can process multiple inputs, using multiple modalities when presenting material can enhance their understanding. Third, keeping interactions brief maximizes comprehension, attention, and recall of information. For example, therapists can use concrete, one-step requests rather than multi-step requests when giving instructions. Fourth, repetition may be necessary to help persons with brain injury who have concentration, memory, or language difficulties. Finally, they may need extra time to process information or requests, and thus therapists may need to provide them with more time to answer.

Helping persons with brain injury reduce memory problems can have a positive effect on their behavior. Having an environment that provides cues can help with recall, depending on the type of memory problems they have. For example, verbal cues may assist them in completing activities or remembering information. Written cues, such as putting their names on their door, or pictorial cues, such as posting personal photos in specific locations, can help them compensate for orientation, pathfinding, or memory problems. Calendars, clocks, and watches cue them to the date and time. Use of a memory book or appointment book is a memory cue for many persons with brain injury. Those individuals with brain injury who have good executive abilities may find an electronic date book (i.e., a PDA [personal data assistant]) to be an effective memory aid as well as an organizational tool. Finally, providing information in smaller, more manageable amounts can also be an effective approach in assisting with organization and memory tasks.

Hallucinations/delusions

Hallucinations occur when persons with brain injury experience distorted perceptions. The American Psychiatric Association indicates that hallucinations may occur in any sensory modality: visual, auditory, olfactory, tactile, or gustatory.[1] They may be benign, such as seeing a child sitting under a tree in the back yard. More frequently, however, hallucinations tend to be disturbing and negative in nature. Delusions are erroneous beliefs that often involve misinterpretation of perceptions or experiences.[1] Brain injury can lead to delusions because of the damage to the brain's ability to accurately perceive information. Commonly, delusions are persecutory, grandiose, religious, referential, or somatic in nature, or they may entail the belief that someone is in love with the individual.[1] Paranoid ideation is another feature that can accompany hallucinations and delusions. When these symptoms occur, it is important for nonphysician therapists to inform the team psychiatrist or other physicians.

There are several interventions that therapists can use when persons with brain injury display hallucinations. (See Table 5.13 for the core plan.) An environment can be created in which therapists are available to listen to the persons and acknowledge their feelings about their perceptions. This can have a calming effect. Therapists can attempt to gently redirect them to the current setting or the task at hand. When they are too preoccupied with the hallucination or delusion to respond to redirection, therapists may want to try to orient them to reality in a non-confrontational manner, but only when they are not agitated by reorientation and when therapists have good rapport with them. In the case of agitated persons with brain injury or when good rapport does not exist, therapists should delete this intervention from the plan to prevent escalation to aggressiveness. Occasionally, therapists can be effective by interventions within the hallucinatory scheme. For example, when a person with brain injury thinks the room is flooding a therapist can go over to the bathroom and make a display of turning off the water.

Therapists can also address underlying issues that seem to be related to the delusions of persons with brain injury by exploration of alternative coping strategies: problem solving, social skills training, self-esteem

Table 5.13 Hallucinations/Delusions

Interventions
1. Listen to and acknowledge person's feelings about their perceptions. Provide reassurance.
2. Gently redirect to current setting or task.
3. Orient to reality in non-confrontational manner.
4. Explore alternative coping strategies with person based on cognitive abilities (e.g., problem solving, social skills training, self-esteem improvement strategies, or relationship skills training).
5. Follow through on any promises made to decrease person's suspiciousness.
6. Assist in compensating for memory deficits to reduce misinterpretations.

improvement strategies, and interpersonal relationship skills training (such as the ability to trust others). These approaches can be helpful if the persons with brain injury have the cognitive capacity to learn skills or benefit from insight work.

The neuropsychosocial approach can also assist persons with brain injury who tend to have paranoid ideation. It is important to spend time listening to them in order to build an environment of rapport and trust. It is equally necessary for therapists to follow through on any promises that they make and to be clear about what they can and cannot do when attempting to gain trust. Therapists can begin to question the negative assumptions of persons with brain injury and offer alternative reasons for others' behavior or for why events have occurred. In addition, therapists can address memory deficits that may underlie paranoia. Therapists can observe this when suspiciousness arises from inaccurate recall of events and subsequent misinterpretation of other peoples' motives, but such interventions will likely be ineffective if therapists have not first gained the trust of the person with brain injury. When delusions persist, therapists must consider whether the person with brain injury presents a risk of exhibiting self-injurious behavior or aggression toward others. Therapists can then implement behavior plans for those behaviors.

Social withdrawal

Social withdrawal occurs when persons with brain injury have at least some capacity to interact with others, yet isolate. (See Table 5.14 for the core plan.) Many people enjoy quiet time alone; this is both healthy and socially accepted. However, it is considered unusual when people spend all or nearly all their time alone when not engaged in any specific activity. Persons with brain injury may demonstrate this behavior because of depression and feeling uncomfortable or scared in a new setting. In addition, because of language or cognitive deficits, persons with brain injury who have not yet adjusted to their deficits may be unsure of how to interact with others in a new way. They may have poor awareness of their deficits and may not feel that they need to be in a treatment setting or in a supervised living setting.

Table 5.14 Social Withdrawal

	Interventions
1.	Offer person frequent opportunities for socialization.
2.	Assist person in gradually integrating into social situations or create environment where person can socialize individually.
3.	Structure treatment and daily activities to utilize leisure interests.
4.	Provide daily schedule as needed.
5.	If person is depressed, provide emotional support and arrange for psychotherapy based on person's cognitive abilities.
6.	Provide rationale for treatment if person shows poor awareness of deficits.

Therefore, they may isolate themselves because they perceive themselves to have nothing in common with others in that setting.

Several interventions can reduce social withdrawal. Therapists can create an environment in which persons with brain injury who exhibit social withdrawal can gradually integrate into social situations. For example, by allowing them to sit on the outskirts of a group and not expecting them to respond to questions or interact initially, persons with brain injury may feel more comfortable and confident about participating over time. At a later date, they may be able to join the group and show increased participation. These persons may also be most successful behaviorally if they can maintain a low participation role. Alternatively, therapists may structure their world so that they can socialize individually and their environment does not require group interaction.

Sometimes persons with brain injury withdraw because they are depressed. (Treatment strategies for depression appear in the plan for suicidal/depressive statements.) They may feel uncomfortable being around other people with brain injury, and therefore avoid interactions with them. The more comfortable they become with their own brain injury and its impact on their functioning, the more comfortable they are likely to feel around other persons with brain injury. Therapists can explore with them what would make them more comfortable and structure interactions that permit a greater degree of comfort. For example, they may feel more at ease with other persons with brain injury at a similar level of function to their own.

When persons with brain injury have the ability to gain from them, traditional methods of intervention can also be in the therapists' armamentarium. Psychotherapy, education, and social skills training can assist with emotional adjustment. Rehabilitation therapies can help improve their abilities and help them learn to compensate for residual cognitive and language deficits that may impact social withdrawal.

In regard to withdrawal from treatment, some persons with brain injury have poor awareness of their brain injury and of the need to interact with others in treatment. Giving them a rationale for the purpose of therapies or their treatment plan and involving them in the planning of these activities tends to increase participation. Providing them with daily schedules helps them plan and recall expectations. Structuring their treatment plan to utilize their interests can improve the amount of their social interaction. They may laugh, talk with others, and put forth great effort when therapy can incorporate their interests. For example, during communication skills therapy a person who generally does not speak to others may participate when the topic therapists use to work on communication is horses, because of a pre-morbid love of riding.

Noncompliance

Noncompliance results when persons with brain injury do not follow the requests or the recommendations of their therapists. (See Table 5.15 for the

Table 5.15 Noncompliance

Interventions
1. Assess person's reason for not engaging in activity by directly asking them.
2. Acknowledge person's thoughts and feelings. Attempt to resolve issues person raises.
3. If ineffective, educate about purpose and benefits of activity and about results and risks of noncompliance.
4. Eliminate nonessential demands that person does not comply with.
5. Negotiate with person, based on cognitive abilities.
6. Seek out alternative solutions (e.g., complete cares in afternoon if person refuses morning cares).
7. Provide a written schedule of daily activities and a list of medications person is prescribed and their uses.
8. Give brief verbal reminders prior to an activity.
9. Integrate person's leisure interests into daily activities.

core plan.) Noncompliance may take the form of refusal to take medications, go to therapies or doctor's appointments, eat or drink, get up from bed or go to sleep, go to work or to other daily activities, participate in leisure activities, or complete daily cares. This behavior can create feelings of frustration, anger, and helplessness in those around them. However, therapists who ground their approach in neuropsychosocial treatment methods can implement interventions to reduce noncompliance.

The first intervention in the core behavior plan for noncompliance is to assess the reasons for noncompliance by talking with persons with brain injury about the activity they refuse to participate in and asking them directly why they do not want to engage in it. It is important to acknowledge their thoughts and feelings if they are able to articulate their reasons for noncompliance. They may comply with the activity once therapists attempt to resolve the reasons identified as the cause of noncompliance. However, if the noncompliance continues therapists should provide education about the purpose and potential benefits of treatment or the activity that is refused and provide information about the results and potential risks of noncompliant behavior.

Therapists need to consider whether there is any risk of not complying if persons with brain injury continue to refuse the treatment or activity. Therapists should respect their choice if it does not cause harm to the persons with brain injury or others. It is important to avoid a power struggle, particularly over noncompliance with a nonessential activity. In the neuropsychosocial approach, therapists should consider elimination of nonessential demands when persons with brain injury fail to comply. When the dynamic of a power struggle disappears, persons with brain injury may choose to do an activity or follow a treatment plan independently. Negotiating with persons with brain injury when possible is essential to avoid power struggles that may increase their feelings of resistance to doing an activity that others desire them to do. However, negotiation is unrealistic for some persons with severe cognitive deficits who are unable to use negotiation skills.

Therapists should look for alternative solutions to noncompliance. For example, when persons with brain injury refuse to complete their morning cares despite discussions of the purposes and benefits of cares and resulting problems of refusing cares, therapists may find that they are able to complete cares later in the day. Therefore, a creative solution is to structure the environment to allow completion of cares at an alternative time.

There are other changes therapists can make in the world of persons with brain injury to address noncompliance. Providing a written schedule of daily treatments or activities can improve participation. Writing out information about medications and their uses can help improve medication compliance. Giving brief verbal reminders prior to an activity can assist persons with memory and initiation problems. Assessing the leisure interests of persons with brain injury and then utilizing them in therapies can increase participation. Persons with brain injury who love music but display resistance to going to therapy, for instance, may initiate more in therapy when therapists play music in the background or when therapists use something relating to music as a treatment task.

Several interventions can be added to the core behavior plan for noncompliance. Therapists should base these interventions on the reasons for the noncompliance and the specific type of noncompliant behavior that persons with brain injury exhibit. Sometimes medication noncompliance is based upon fear of side effects or misunderstandings about the purposes of the medications. Therapists can structure the world of persons with brain injury to include scheduled opportunities for them to speak with the physician who has prescribed the medications. Persons with brain injury may show enhanced compliance when they know that therapists routinely inform their physicians of their specific physical complaints that might be side effects. Therapists can create an environment in which persons with brain injury are more comfortable in taking their medications.

Persons with brain injury will at times refuse to attend physician appointments, therapies, work, day program, or leisure activities. The reasons for refusals may include depressed mood, unawareness of deficit, and fatigue. Therapists should see core behavior plans for depression and unawareness of deficit to treat these causes of refusal. Fatigue may be a factor if persons with brain injury have trouble sleeping at night and therefore are unable to function sufficiently to participate in these activities during daytime hours. Treating sleep problems can improve alertness, and ultimately compliance. Medications can aid with sleep. (See Chapter 6 for a discussion of medication use.) Good sleep habits, too, are important.

Persons with brain injury may refuse to eat or drink. Therapists can change the environment of eating by manipulation of the type, amount, schedule, or presentation of food or drink. One way to improve intake is to consider the food preferences of those persons who refuse food or drink. It is helpful to have a dietician visit with them and make recommendations. Observing and documenting what foods they eat is particularly necessary with persons who are unable to verbalize their preferences due to aphasia or cognitive impairment. Another strategy is to present one type of food at a time or small amounts of food to decrease the tendency of some persons with brain injury to become overwhelmed when they face a plate full of food. It may also help to assist them to begin eating. They may have initiation problems, but will continue to eat a meal after therapists assist them with getting started. A further approach is to include finger food, if tactile sensations help overcome taste and smell impairments. Persons with brain injury often accept flavored drink supplements more easily than other food or drink, but these supplements need to be ordered by a physician. Refusal to eat or drink can be serious and even life threatening if left untreated. If persons with brain injury exhibit noncompliance with eating or drinking, medical consultation is necessary. Such noncompliance may reflect a medical etiology requiring medical evaluation. This behavior may also be due to other causes, such as depression or a premorbid eating disorder, that therapists should factor into treatment.

Therapists sometimes misperceive persons with brain injury as being noncompliant when in fact they are displaying cognitive deficits. Persons with memory problems may forget to go to their appointments or take their medication. If they are disoriented they may refuse to get out of bed or to go to therapy. Structuring their environment to help them compensate for their cognitive deficits will improve their level of participation.

Unawareness/denial of deficit

Unawareness or denial of one's cognitive or physical problems are common sequelae following brain injury. (See Table 5.16 for the core plan.) Persons with brain injury who have anasognosia (an organic unawareness of deficits) or denial (emotional hurdles interfering with acceptance) often present with more challenges than their counterparts who have awareness of their deficits. Those who have awareness and insight into their deficits are often able to apply their residual strengths and compensate for their deficits, which improves their overall functioning. This improvement in overall functioning, in turn, has a profoundly positive effect on their emotional status and behavioral control. Conversely, persons with brain injury who show unawareness or denial of deficits have more trouble applying their strengths and compensating for their weaknesses, which ultimately effects their emotional status and behavioral control in a negative manner. Hence, poor behavioral control and unawareness or denial of deficits often occur together. This combination leads to persons with brain injury engaging in dyscontrol, such as driving a vehicle despite therapists identifying their inability to drive.

The first intervention of the core behavior plan for unawareness of deficit is to assess the nature and degree of individuals' unawareness of their deficits. It is helpful to know which specific deficits persons with brain injury are unaware of, as this can impact the type of problems they will have in their everyday functioning. If they are unaware of their physical deficits, they may be at risk for falling. If swallowing problems put them at risk for

Table 5.16 Unawareness/Denial of Deficit

Interventions
1. Assess and document nature and degree of unawareness of deficits.
2. Gently confront person by verbally identifying deficit in a relaxed, brief, concrete manner.
3. Normalize deficits by providing education about brain injury.
4. Offer opportunities to participate in activities in safe conditions that demonstrate strengths and deficits.
5. Monitor for depressed, angry, or anxious mood if awareness improves.
6. Provide emotional support and identify cognitive compensatory strategies and ways to apply strengths as awareness improves.
7. When awareness remains limited, structure environment around person to increase safety (e.g., provide necessary supervision; provide locked facility; pursue conservatorship; remove and prevent access to car keys, vehicles, firearms, motorized tools, sharp objects and alcohol or illicit drugs).
8. In treating psychological denial, address emotional needs as slowly expose person to deficits over time.

aspiration, they may sneak food to eat and develop pneumonia. If they are unaware of their cognitive deficits, they may attempt to engage in activities that are unsafe or at which they fail, such as: driving, using motorized tools, living alone, self administering medications, taking alcohol or illicit drugs, using firearms, or returning to a previous vocation or school beyond their abilities.

The next intervention in the core behavior plan is to gently confront individuals who demonstrate unawareness when they are calm by verbally identifying a deficit. Identifying a deficit is most effective if feedback is given in a relaxed, brief, concrete, and direct manner. Repetition is generally necessary to help them recognize the deficit as well as to generalize how it may impact other aspects of their lives. Because persons with brain injury tend to rely on their own perception of reality rather than that of others, it is important for therapists to provide them with opportunities to participate in activities in safe conditions toward the goal of improved awareness. It is also important to recognize that the level of emotional distress experienced by persons with brain injury often increases as awareness of their deficits improves. The result can be increased depression, anger, or anxiety. Therefore, persons with brain injury will probably benefit from extra emotional and social support as they become more aware of their deficits, as well as from assistance in identifying cognitive compensatory strategies and ways to apply their cognitive strengths.

Many persons with brain injury do not respond to these approaches, and their awareness remains impaired. Some persons may exhibit improved awareness temporarily when they are confronted with a deficit, yet this improved awareness may not carry over beyond the immediate moment. Others may acknowledge deficits in their cognition, yet be unable to generalize how these would impact their functional abilities such as need for supervision, assistance with decision making, or not being able to drive. This lack of awareness often results in subsequent behavior problems. The focus of treatment for persons with these difficulties is to structure the environment around them to help them function optimally.

Therapists need to develop a neuropsychosocial plan to ensure the safest environment for the persons with brain injury and others around them. The following are some ways in which therapists can adjust the environment to increase safety: providing supervision commensurate with the risk their unawareness produces (from phone check-in to 24-hour supervision); providing a locked facility; pursuing conservatorship for medical and/or personal decision making; preventing access to car keys and vehicles; removing firearms from the home and making access to firearms impossible; removing motorized tools from the home as well as access to them; preventing access to sharp or potentially dangerous objects such as straight razors; creating an environment free of alcohol or illicit drugs; and removing access to medications when appropriate. Therapists will expand this list as needed based upon the risks of various environments and the associated unawareness of the inability to manage those items or activities.

Some persons with brain injury do have awareness of deficits. This awareness may trigger a painful emotional process that they attempt to cope with through psychological denial of their deficits or of necessary restrictions. The approach to treatment for psychological denial contrasts with that for treating organic unawareness, outlined above. In treating psychological denial, the environmental support for decreased defensiveness is crucial. The emotional need to maintain denial must be addressed by the environment so that acknowledgment of deficits can grow as therapists slowly expose persons with brain injury to their deficits over time. Nevertheless, some persons with brain injury are unable to overcome their denial. In such cases, therapists need to apply a neuropsychosocial approach similar to the one they use when unawareness of deficit persists.

Socially inappropriate behavior

Socially inappropriate behaviors are actions that others view as offensive in nature. (See Table 5.17 for the core plan.) They are acts that other people perceive as offensive because they violate societal norms beyond merely being behaviors or a style that is unique or unusual. Mild to moderate socially inappropriate behaviors relate to social pragmatic difficulties such as saying things in an offensive way, having poor timing, talking or laughing too loudly or too long, repeating oneself, singing or humming repeatedly or in public, snapping one's fingers repeatedly at others, carrying small animals with oneself everywhere, or making obscene gestures. Another type of socially inappropriate behavior includes intrusive behaviors, which includes asking personal questions of therapists or strangers, sharing personal information with strangers, standing too close to others, and touching others in a non-sexual yet inappropriate manner. An additional set of specific

Table 5.17 Socially Inappropriate Behavior

Interventions
1. Label behavior in a non-judgmental manner.
2. Redirect or distract away from subject or object.
3. Create low stimulation environment.
4. Prevent disinhibited behaviors by preparing person for novel, complex or stimulating activities (e.g., break activity down into concrete steps to follow, provide rehearsal, repetition, and written information about steps).
5. Model appropriate behavior by maintaining good physical boundaries and identifying roles in relationships.
6. Develop with person concrete cues to redirect inappropriate behavior (e.g., arms length distance, a facial expression, a short phrase, or lines on floor).
7. Provide positive attention for socially acceptable behaviors.
8. Attempt other strategies if person responds negatively to direct feedback (e.g., use humor, ignore inappropriate behaviors, or first provide praise and then identify behavior).
9. Respond to behaviors that have attention seeking component with flat affect and neutral tone of voice. Avoid verbalizations and strong emotional response.
10. Avoid situations in which person has shown inappropriate behavior in the past.

behaviors considered socially inappropriate by most people is poor hygiene. Poor hygiene includes not changing bedding, not cleaning one's room or personal living area, leaving perishable food out to spoil, not showering or changing clothes to the point of developing body odor, not washing one's hands after becoming soiled with feces, and not wearing adult incontinence products or changing clothes despite bowel or bladder incontinence. Other socially unacceptable behaviors are more severe, such as smearing or eating feces.

The first intervention of the core behavior plan for socially inappropriate behavior is to label the behavior in a non-judgmental manner. Persons with brain injury may be unaware that the behavior is offensive, irritating, or unacceptable to others. Giving them this social feedback creates awareness that the world finds their behavior unacceptable. When labeling alone is ineffective in discontinuing the behavior, use of redirection or distraction can shift the person's attention off the inappropriate behavior. Therapists may institute a low-stimulation environment, because overstimulation increases disinhibition and the likelihood of inappropriate behavior, while a low-stimulation environment decreases the probability of socially inappropriate behavior.

Cognitive deficits can affect socially inappropriate behavior. Therapists can treat the cognitive deficits that impact inappropriate behavior by altering the environment. They can set up the availability of supportive people who will be available to persons with brain injury to identify ways to manage situations in which they have been inappropriate in the past. Such people can talk about any novel, complex, or stimulating activity ahead of time and break the activity down into concrete steps that can reduce disinhibited behaviors. Discussing potential unexpected events that may occur and how persons with brain injury can deal with them prior to an event is helpful. Providing rehearsal, repetition, and written information about the steps to follow helps persons with brain injury anticipate and organize their thoughts so that they are better able to manage novel or complex situations. Finally, therapists can prohibit persons with brain injury from returning to situations in which they have shown inappropriate behavior in the past.

Sometimes, despite awareness of social norms, persons with brain injury may find it extremely difficult to inhibit their impulses in social situations. The approach of utilizing their interests when planning social activities can motivate them to put forth the effort that may help them to inhibit their behavior somewhat, even if for only a short period of time. When this intervention fails to eliminate inappropriate behaviors, therapists should either avoid creating situations in which persons with brain injury engage in socially inappropriate behavior or make adjustments to the surroundings. For example, some persons may make offensive comments to others in large groups, but show less offensive behavior in small groups. In these cases, the neuropsychosocial environment would entail social activity in small groups.

Higher-level cognitive and social pragmatic difficulties can underlie socially inappropriate behavior. If persons with brain injury have trouble accurately reading nonverbal cues and either miss or misinterpret the cues, they may act inappropriately. They also may display nonverbal gestures incongruent with their emotions, which results in their sending the wrong message. Consequently, they may display behaviors that are out of step with the rest of the group or not in line with the conversation. The more pronounced and public such errors, the more disruptive they are to others. Occasionally, persons with brain injury can benefit if therapists teach them social pragmatic skills; however, they may need to avoid certain settings when skill building fails or have therapists put in place neuropsychosocial cues for them.

Therapists can develop some simple concrete neuropsychosocial cues to redirect persons with brain injury when they display inappropriate behavior. These cues are effective when the behavior has previously been identified and discussed with them. Persons with brain injury, for example, may verbally agree to work on avoiding a behavior, but have trouble inhibiting it. A case in point is when persons with poor boundaries repeatedly touch therapists. Therapists can provide them with a concrete cue by holding their arm out to indicate the physical distance that they need to respect during their conversations. Persons with brain injury who have previously agreed to this limit will generally respond to this redirection. A certain facial expression or look from therapists can remind them of the limit. A short phrase, lyrics from a song, a private joke, or a visual image can also suffice as cues. For example, one image that has been helpful for some people who are physically intrusive is that of a bubble that exists around others that they cannot touch or it will break. In addition, a rule that they must be 4 feet from other people during conversations can be effective. Finally, placing lines on the floor to designate areas that are for therapists only or are off-limits can be useful to cue persons with brain injury who have boundary problems.

Therapists should always model appropriate behavior. They should maintain well-defined roles in relationships with persons with brain injury by explaining therapists' purpose for their relationship with them. For example, therapists can clarify for an individual that the purpose of a particular therapy is to help that person learn to walk again, and not to date that individual. They should maintain good physical boundaries by always keeping an arm's length from persons who stand too close to them. They should also model boundaries by setting the norms. For example, with persons who request to shake hands constantly, therapist should only shake hands at the beginning and the end of a session.

Some persons with brain injury judge others to be unreasonably critical when they receive negative feedback about their socially inappropriate behavior. They may respond by ignoring feedback or becoming aggressive. Therapists need to create an environment in which feedback is common and acceptable. Therefore, therapists should first provide praise and then identify inappropriate behavior while providing an alternative way of saying or doing something. Humor, if used effectively, can also be useful in redirecting persons from socially inappropriate behavior. The humor needs to be collaborative in nature, though, so that the persons with brain injury can laugh at therapists and themselves. Otherwise, the use of humor can be demeaning or humiliating. At times it can be useful to simply ignore inappropriate behavior. Therapists must take care to avoid creating an environment that is constantly critical, particularly early in treatment and with persons with brain injury who are assaultive, and to provide praise when persons with brain injury behave in socially acceptable ways.

Hygiene problems are a particularly vexing variant of socially inappropriate behavior among persons with brain injury. A lack of awareness of how their own behavior impacts others often underlies hygiene problems. They may be unable to perceive the necessity of bathing, and as a result do not do so unless cued by others. In these cases, it may be helpful to provide concrete feedback alerting them to the fact that they have an odor that is offensive to others. They may still need verbal cueing from others or a written schedule to help them remember to follow through. Some persons with brain injury may even need direct step-by-step cueing to complete each hygiene task in a thorough manner, even though they do not need actual physical assistance with these tasks. Some persons with brain injury may refuse to complete these tasks as a way to assert their sense of control. Therapists can address this situation by creating a world for these persons where it is relatively acceptable if they choose to bathe less frequently. For example, these persons will need to stay away from public places such as shopping malls or restaurants, and avoid social gatherings. When presented with these choices, some persons with brain injury often choose to improve their hygiene despite their reduced awareness of the need for hygiene. However, others may choose to avoid social situations and comply with minimal but medically acceptable hygiene standards.

Some of the more severe socially unacceptable behaviors such as smearing or eating feces often have an attention-seeking component. In the case of persons with brain injury who are continent, other similar behaviors are urinating in public places or in odd places. These behaviors may be an expression of anger toward therapists or toward themselves or may be an acting-out behavior by persons with brain injury who are depressed. Other people may inadvertently encourage these behaviors by their strong response to them. For example, a woman with brain injury puts her own feces in her mouth in the common area on a hospital unit. Therapists and other patients respond strongly with disgust conveyed through verbalizations, sighs, facial expression, tone of voice, and a quick response to the behavior. The woman perceives the strong response and therefore continues the behavior. The treatment approach in this case is to immediately manage the situation while avoiding giving the individual social attention for the behavior. Therapists can do this by keeping a flat affect, avoiding verbalizations or sighs, and by speaking in a neutral tone of voice. They then can give the person short and concrete requests such as, "Please spit it out," and place a towel beneath her mouth. Beyond such immediate interventions, it is important to include scheduled times for social attention in her environment to ensure that the individual is receiving enough attention for appropriate behavior.

Anxiety

Anxiety refers to the internal feelings of arousal or fear experienced by persons with brain injury that result in disruptive behaviors. (See Table 5.18 for the core plan.) These behaviors may be in the form of compulsive, repetitive, or ritualistic behaviors such as repetitive hand washing; rituals during dressing, cares, or eating; excessive or uncontrolled crying; aggression; attempts to elope; or non-compliance, to name a few. Previous core behavior plans for aggression, attempts to elope, and non-compliance suggest ways to treat anxiety resulting in these behaviors. Persons experiencing anxiety may also engage in self-injurious behavior such as persistent scratching or picking at themselves, which is dealt with in the plan for self-injurious behavior.

The first intervention in the core behavior plan for anxiety is to assess the triggers. Some examples of triggers are a visit from someone, an altercation with another person, or being in an unfamiliar environment. Common environmental triggers include noise level and the overall level of stimulation.

Therapists may begin treatment with the traditional approaches of desensitization or by teaching coping skills to reduce anxiety such as relaxation training, anger management, assertiveness training, or problem solving. As always, therapists need to modify these approaches to fit the

Table 5.18 Anxiety

Interventions
1. Assess triggers for anxiety.
2. Redirect or distract to another topic or activity.
3. If effective, offer person opportunities to verbally express feelings.
4. Provide concrete, simple solutions.
5. Model calm behavior and provide reassurance.
6. Use simple written reassurances when person requires more constant assistance.
7. Alter physical environment to prevent person from harming self (e.g., move bed away from wall if person repeatedly bangs head against wall when anxious).

cognitive level of persons with brain injury, typically by keeping material concrete and brief, and by reminding persons with brain injury to use the skills. However, therapists commonly find that these traditional approaches need to be supplemented by the neuropsychosocial approach.

In this regard, therapists should first attempt redirection or distraction when persons with brain injury engage in anxious behaviors. When this is not effective, the environment should include opportunities for them to verbally express their feelings to reduce behaviors. This should include having therapists available to provide concrete, simple solutions to problems, since persons with brain injury may have trouble generating solutions. In addition, they can model calm behavior and provide reassurance. Simple written reassurances may assist some persons who either have memory problems or require more constant reassurance. In this vein, it may be important for persons with brain injury who have more severe impairment to have therapists wear nametags that provide identification. In brief, in many cases therapists can decrease anxiety by making sure that persons with brain injury can readily identify in their environment therapeutic resources that will provide emotional support and solve problems.

Changing the physical environment to help prevent persons with brain injury from harming themselves is the most prudent approach to follow for severe behavior. For example, some persons repeatedly bang their head against the rails of their bed when they are anxious. Considering physical changes such as placing pads on the rails or making sure the bed is not near a wall or other hard surface can reduce the risk of harm. In such cases, therapists can refer to the plan for self-injurious behaviors.

One possible change to the core behavior plan for anxiety would be to avoid informing persons with brain injury of potentially stressful events in advance when they experience anticipatory anxiety that leads to behavioral problems. It may be best in this type of situation to tell them about an event just prior to its occurrence rather than too far in advance. Conversely, other persons may show a reduction in anxiety when they know information about an event ahead of time and thus may display fewer problem behaviors. Determining which approach to use must be based on careful observation and assessment of responses to previous approaches. One final addition to the plan is to avoid giving persons too many decisions to make when they have trouble with decision making.

Conclusions

How do therapists apply the neuropsychosocial approach? The key to this approach is the development and implementation of written behavior plans. First, therapists need to identify target behaviors and initiate core behavior plans to address the problem behaviors. Throughout the course of treatment, therapists need to customize the behavior plan. Ultimately, they create a plan for each individual with brain injury that identifies how to alter that person's physical environment and indicates how others can maximize the person's behavioral control and functional abilities. Traditional approaches can sometimes be useful, but when they prove insufficient, therapists can institute a neuropsychosocial intervention plan.

A solid understanding of the underpinnings or phenomenology of the behavior problems of persons with brain injury is essential in developing interventions that accurately treat their behavior. The core behavior plan to treat a behavior problem can change dramatically with additions and deletions based on the underpinnings of the behavior. Therapists need to consider the cognitive strengths and weaknesses of persons with brain injury when determining which interventions are possible to attempt as well as which interventions will be most effective. They need to take into account the level of emotional control and adjustment of each person with brain injury, because these factors also impact the interventions therapists choose and how they deliver them. Therapists' delivery of interventions, such as their tone of voice and affect, are often as important as the actual interventions. In fact, the way in which therapists deliver material to persons with brain injury can be an intervention in the behavior plan itself.

Flexibility, creativity, and teamwork are necessary ingredients in the development and implementation of a behavior plan. Therapists need to be flexible enough to change the plan regularly based on the response. They need to be creative and innovate in order to generate interventions that will result in the best outcome for persons with brain injury. They need to avoid becoming too emotionally attached to any one approach, since it may not be the ultimate answer. Teamwork is paramount in creating, altering, and implementing behavior plans. Consistency of the plan is equally crucial, and excellent communication is necessary to achieve this goal.

Creating, adapting, and implementing behavior plans is a challenging task. However, it can be extremely rewarding work as therapists expand their skills and conceptual horizons to produce an effective plan. It is very satisfying to help persons with brain injury achieve a successful outcome of behavior control through the neuropsychosocial approach.

Reference

1. *Diagnostic and Statistical Manual of Mental Disorders*, 4th Ed., American Psychiatric Association, Washington, D.C., 1994, 275.

chapter six

The role of medications in behavioral management

Robert Sevenich

Introduction

Medication management in persons with brain injury offers unique challenges for the health care delivery system and for physicians. Major advancements in intensive care allow many people whose injuries would have been fatal in the past to survive. Unfortunately, treatment for the resultant cognitive, emotional, and behavioral difficulties for persons with brain injury continues to be a major challenge in health care, and research in this area is still in its infancy.

The medical community does not yet have an adequate understanding of normal brain function, and has even less understanding of dysfunction of the damaged brain. The brain is a complex organ, intricately interwoven with various neurochemical transmitters for which new subsets are being discovered as researchers probe its physiology. Knowledge of how the various neurochemicals interact with one another is still rudimentary. Although even a small lesion in a single area of the brain may have profound effects on chemical pathways and affect the functioning in other areas of the brain, it is not clear how or why. Most information about neurochemical function as it relates to behavior comes from general psychiatry and neurology. Yet, many theories and much of our current knowledge may not be readily applicable to the damaged brain.

Due to the difficulty with pharmacological management of this population, repeated or prolonged psychiatric hospitalizations due to behavioral dyscontrol are common for persons with brain injury. Aggression, perhaps the most difficult target symptom to manage, is a frequent reason for loss of community placement. Assaults on therapists or on other persons with brain injury occurring in the hospital setting are commonly the result of organic brain dysfunction.[1] Yet, the current mental health system is not well equipped to serve these persons.

Although psychiatrists frequently are asked to manage the emotional and behavioral sequelae that often follow brain injury, neurologists, internists, family practitioners, and many other specialists often are consulted to address these difficult issues. It is essential that these physicians have a treatment approach for medication management of behavioral dyscontrol by persons with brain injury. Also, they must remember that the goal for treating persons with brain injury should be to maximize independence by improving cognition while decreasing aggression and other aspects of behavioral dyscontrol.

Clinical challenges

Many reasons exist for the challenges in treating behavioral dyscontrol in persons with brain injury. In other areas of medicine, appropriate diagnosis dictates treatment protocol. The challenge for physicians usually exists in making the appropriate diagnosis. After diagnosis, treatment protocols have a predictive success rate. The diagnosis of brain injury, however, lacks a consistent and clinically relevant nomenclature. *The Diagnostic and Statistical Manual-IV* (DSM-IV) does define the diagnostic criteria for Dementia Due to Brain Injury.[2] This diagnosis exists as a subset of the Diagnostic Criteria for Dementia Due to Other General Medical Conditions. It recognizes the variety of cognitive, emotional, and behavioral sequelae due to brain injury but does little to categorize the symptoms into treatment-relevant groupings, and offers little to aid physicians in treatment options. In addition, absent an underlying or comorbid reversible medical problem, radiographic and laboratory data offer little treatment guidance. Unfortunately, the traditional medical model fails to offer guidance to physicians.

Hence, appropriate definition and quantifying of actual behavioral difficulties becomes extremely difficult. Persons with brain injury can have a wide array of clinical presentations and often appear refractory to standard psychiatric medications. This population varies greatly in its responses to traditional treatment modalities. Physicians must not assume that persons with brain injury will have a clinical course or response to treatment that parallels other psychiatric diagnoses. Much of the frustration and accompanying poor outcomes that occur when providing treatment of this population can be attributed to physicians' expectations of a treatment response based on their experience with the general psychiatric population.

Perhaps the most important consideration in addressing physical aggression in persons with brain injury is to understand the underlying phenomenology of the behaviors (See Chapter 4). Physicians must look at the underlying cognitive or emotional deficits that drove a particular behavior. Persons with brain injury may punch a hole in the wall because they are frustrated, depressed, impulsive, or even psychotic. They may have an anxiety disorder driven by obsessional or paranoid thoughts and impulse control difficulties which led to the behavior. Identifying the precursors to the behavior will help identify the phenomenology of dyscontrol and is very important when addressing a multi-modality approach in diminishing such behavior.

In addition to difficulties regarding definition and diagnosis, how persons with brain injury present themselves often represents a roadblock for physicians. Persons with brain injury are often unreliable historians, and this complicates treatment. Many have severed ties with family and other caregivers, so collateral sources of information may be lacking. Issues of chemical dependency often make treatment more complex and may increase the risks associated with the variety of medication choices available to physicians. Organic and psychological denial are also common.[3] Physicians often face defiance as they help persons with brain injury realize that they have difficulties and that treatment is warranted. Many of these persons expect to go back to their lives prior to the brain injury and will not accept environmental modifications, restrictions on their independence, or medications to manage emotional difficulties.

All of these issues make the development of rapport with persons with brain injury extremely challenging. Physicians, however, should not be discouraged with lack of patient participation and rapport development early in the treatment course, as persons with brain injury often require a substantial amount of time in coming to the realization that they need assistance and medication. Even if persons with brain injury terminate contact with their physicians, the physicians should leave an "open door" for them to be able to return in a way that will limit the amount of embarrassment upon return.

Treatment compliance is often a significant hurdle for care. If their safety is at risk and their judgment is significantly impaired the physician may need to seek the protection of the court for the person with brain injury, with the court imposing treatment. Civil commitment may be the only avenue for many of them to enter treatment. Unfortunately, the protection of the court is often viewed as coercion or punishment; this perception, in turn, can increase resistance and diminish rapport. Even in such situations, physicians should try to offer persons with brain injury as much control over certain decisions as possible. Encouraging persons with brain injury to make decisions regarding appointment times, appropriate activities, topics for discussion during the interview, and even specific timing of dosages provides them with an increased sense of control and self-dignity, thus improving rapport.

For treatment to be successful, it must be individualized for each person according to the set of target symptoms presented. Medication decisions and trials need to be done in the context of a broader overall neuropsychosocial treatment plan. Respect for the individual's autonomy, to the degree possible, is paramount in promoting treatment success. Finally, there must be good communication between the various therapists and physicians for a positive outcome.

This treatment approach recognizes the importance of improvement in quality of life. Too often, the decrease in maladaptive or aggressive behaviors occurs at the expense of cognitive and physical functioning. Given the perception that there are no other options, many physicians, therapists, and health care systems will accept over-sedation as a necessary outcome of pharmacological control of aggression. Elimination of maladaptive behaviors cannot be the single goal for treatment. Physicians must try to also maximize the cognitive and functional ability of persons with brain injury in order to achieve improvements in quality of life. Stability or even improvement in the area of functional independence should accompany a decline in the maladaptive target symptoms.

Treatment approach

Physicians must implement a systematic and organized approach when addressing medication management. They should be cognizant of the following three areas of concern:

1. Proper identification of specific target symptoms
2. Consideration of underlying co-existing medical problems including iatrogenic sources
3. Design and implementation of non-pharmacological approaches

Symptom identification

It is imperative for physicians to accurately identify target symptoms before embarking on medication intervention. Accurate identification entails having a careful history supported by collateral sources, since many persons with brain injury have significant deficits in memory or their perceptions of their behavioral dyscontrol make the information they provide about their own behavior unreliable. Furthermore, fear of losing independence or becoming reliant on a medication regime frequently has an impact on their willingness to provide accurate information. Even when there is community supervision it can be difficult to obtain accurate collateral information, because many persons with brain injury residing in supervised settings often present to physicians' clinics either unattended or with little or no clinically relevant documentation.

For this reason, accurate tracking of target symptoms should be a requirement of appropriately supervised residences. The clinical supervisors and direct care therapists of such institutions should receive appropriate education and training on tracking target symptoms. In addition, behavioral tracking sheets or other attempts to objectify behavioral data are beneficial. Otherwise, physicians are forced to rely on the qualitative information gathering and reflection by therapists who are insufficiently familiar with the persons with brain injury to make accurate reports of behavioral incidents or who may have limited access to information about persons with brain injury over time or in different situations. A behavioral tracking methodology provides therapists with a means to convey information in a precise, comprehensive, and helpful fashion. Accurate and objective longitudinal information will help guide physicians in developing an appropriate medication regime.

Neuropsychological test data is also beneficial for physicians as they identify the underlying etiology or phenomenology of the target symptom and make specific medication choices. For example, if target symptoms are at least in part due to significant memory problems, physicians may want to avoid medications that would tend to have a negative impact on memory such as benzodiazepine or anticholinergic agents. In summary, accurate target symptom identification through precise data gathering combined with neuropsychological data is essential prior to embarking on a medication trial.

Co-existing medical problems

Common scenarios

Physicians must address whether the target symptoms are a result of underlying medical problems. Co-existing medical difficulties are common in persons with brain injury. Persons with brain injury often have significant cognitive or behavioral sequelae as a result of comorbid medical conditions or due to the medications used to address those problems.

Early in the recovery period following brain injury, there are often significant co-existing medical issues. Delirium is common in the ICU setting during initial stabilization, but periodic delirium can occur later in the recovery course and can represent a medical emergency that needs immediate attention. Early pain syndromes from headaches and orthopedic injury are also common and may significantly agitate persons with brain injury. Unfortunately, many of the medications used to treat those conditions have a negative impact on cognition and can also cause disinhibition. Management of these situations may require outside medical consultants. Therapists and treating physicians must be aware of the impact of medical problems and iatrogenic medication effects on cognitive, emotional, and behavioral functioning.

Another frequently occurring medical problem that often continues past the period of initial stabilization is seizure disorder. Seizure disorder is common following brain injury. Approximately 20% of survivors of traumatic brain injury with a Glasgow Coma Scale (GCS) score of 10 or lower experience early seizures, and 32% experience at least one late seizure.[4] Subclinical seizures can actually be the etiology of psychotic symptoms and many underlying behavioral disturbances. Proper diagnosis and treatment should involve consultation with neurology.

Chronic pain associated with brain injury and with the orthopedic injuries that often accompany brain injury is also a common medical reason for behavioral dyscontrol. Appropriate pain management techniques are extremely important in this subset of persons with brain injury to improve behavioral control. Unfortunately, many of the medications used for pain control, such as narcotics, may actually increase the amount of aggression and behavioral dyscontrol due to the negative cognitive impact and disinhibition caused by those agents. A referral to a chronic pain specialist who is knowledgeable in treatment of persons with brain injury may be appropriate.

Management processes

Many persons with brain injury see more than one physician. Co-management with other physicians involves attention to the medications each physician prescribes, with vigilance to possible medication interactions and side effects that may exacerbate or even cause the underlying target symptoms. Good communication between multiple prescribers as well as sharing possible treatment suggestions with other specialists is important.

Another important aspect in addressing medical issues for persons with brain injury is constant reassessment of their overall medication regime. Many persons with brain injury have comorbid medical issues that change over time, requiring ongoing medication management, and the medications prescribed for their conditions can often precipitate behavioral dyscontrol, including aggression. Continual assessment of medication interactions, side effects, and necessity is essential. For this reason, a general rule for success when evaluating new persons with brain injury and behavioral dyscontrol is for physicians to minimize or eliminate as many medications as medically appropriate.

It is not uncommon for persons with brain injury, particularly with new onset, to "evolve" over time with regard to their behavioral symptomatology. Attempts at a "medication holiday" if medically appropriate may be warranted to redefine specific target symptoms at various times during their evolution. For example, if attempts at medication management in the community have not been successful in eliminating or curbing maladaptive behaviors such as aggression, especially if symptomatology has worsened, physicians must consider that medications may be at least part of the problem.

Physicians must individualize the decision to initiate a medication holiday for the particular person. In making such a decision, physicians should take into account the potential negative side effects associated with a particular medication regime and the risk of long-term exposure to those medications (such as neuroleptic medication). Physicians may also wish to consider a medication reduction when there has been a change in the person's neuropsychosocial environment that has resulted in more stability, supervision, and oversight. Once the decision for a medication holiday has been made, physicians need to provide for both the safety of the person with brain injury undergoing a medication reduction and that of others. In this regard, slow changes are generally preferable to rapid declines in medication. Decreases in or elimination of certain medications may affect the drug levels of other medications, and the physician must also factor that into the decision. Attempts at significantly decreasing or altering medication may need to be done in a hospital setting to lessen the likelihood of the person becoming aggressive or violent as a result of changes in medication, and to ensure the safety of others. Adding extra therapists to the brain injury unit and strengthening the crisis plan when the treatment entails a medication holiday are wise precautions.

Coordination with non-pharmacological approaches

Prescribing physicians should realize that over time non-pharmacological approaches can be quite successful and may allow persons with brain injury to taper off their use of some or all behavioral medications. Implementation of neuropsychosocial treatment plans can reduce or eliminate the need for behavioral medications. (Of course, a similar decline in behavioral medication usage can occur as a result of the evolution of the brain injury, with improvement in cognitive function and implementation of compensatory strategies.) Even if non-pharmacological approaches have previously been unsuccessful, reattempts at a later point during the clinical course may be warranted. Reinstitution of a non-pharmacological approach further on during the clinical course may be fruitful even if a first attempt was unproductive. If the original disappointing non-pharmacological plan was insight-oriented, skill-building, or contingency management therapy, then the physician should be cognizant of the need to recommend a neuropsychosocial intervention.

While a non-pharmacological approach can mitigate the need for medications, so too can medications enhance a non-pharmacological approach. Persons with brain injury may be more ready to successfully participate in neuropsychosocial interventions after an initial trial of a medication regime. Furthermore, as these persons maintain stability, medications that may have been necessary to control behavior prior to implementing a non-pharmacological approach may no longer be needed and can be reduced or even tapered off.

Again, good communication between physicians and therapists must occur for treatment to be successful. Physicians and therapists must discuss their intent to alter either medication regimes or non-pharmacological plans. If possible, changes in medication and non-pharmacological plans should occur sequentially, not simultaneously. Simultaneous changes increase the number of variables in flux affecting the care. It is often difficult, if not impossible, to attribute an improvement or decline in behavior to a particular change if multiple changes are occurring at the same time.

Medication management for specific target symptoms

It is a considerable challenge for physicians working with persons with brain injury who exhibit behavioral dyscontrol to select effective medications while minimizing side effects. Persons with brain injury may have a higher incidence of adverse effects to medications in general,[5] and this must be taken into account at all times. Thus, the medication choice should be individualized for the specific target symptoms, addressing the phenomenology of those target symptoms and the individual nuances of the person with brain injury. No guide can be all-inclusive. In fact, physicians may develop approaches or use medications not mentioned here which have merit as they determine a particular methodology for particular persons with brain injury. Physicians must use their own judgment and experience while they attend to the idiosyncrasies of each person with brain injury.

Fatigue

Persons with brain injury often struggle with fatigue (mental and physical exhaustion). There are many and varied sources for fatigue. Fatigue may be a result of altered sleep/wake cycles due to the organic insult to the brain.[6] The increase in the cognitive processing and physical effort that persons with brain injury expend to complete tasks may also contribute to fatigue. Typically, persons with brain injury must exert a greater amount of effort and energy in order to perceive, organize, retrieve, and process information. For many, this is an exhausting experience. Other factors can contribute to fatigue as well: chronic pain, gait disturbances, or other mobility and transferring difficulties.

Adequate rest is extremely important for persons with brain injury. Lack of sleep or poor quality of sleep can have enormous implications on cognition as well as mood, and may be the source of or a contributing factor to behavioral dyscontrol. However, many persons with brain injury do not perceive difficulties with sleep. They may have poor recall as to the level of insomnia they are experiencing. Because of this, physicians may need to elicit data from other sources to verify the existence of a sleep problem. Collateral information from spouses, family, or therapists may reveal a previously undiagnosed sleep problem. Tracking sheets or other ways to objectively monitor the sleep patterns of persons with brain injury may also be useful. Physicians should consider conducting a formal sleep study through a sleep center when less intensive monitoring is not helpful.

Persons with brain injury who get 6 to 10 hours of sleep at night may still have inadequate rest. The physical and emotional toll of living with brain injury can easily increase the amount of sleep they need for proper rest relative to their premorbid level of functioning. An increase in behavioral difficulty as the day progresses or following mentally or physically challenging events might suggest fatigue as a possible contributing factor to behavioral dyscontrol. In addition, the clinician should consider injury to the reticular activating system as a potential cause for sleep difficulties.[7]

When addressing a sleep problem, physicians should begin by addressing sleep hygiene. Prior to a trial of a hypnotic agent, they should implement environmental changes that encourage good sleep hygiene. Persons with brain injury should decrease or eliminate their consumption of caffeine, especially after noon; foods such as chocolate and many drinks including colas and tea contain caffeine. In addition, they should avoid alcohol. Physicians and therapists should remind persons with brain injury that even minimal amounts of alcohol, especially in the evening hours, in addition to negatively impacting cognition and behavior, could greatly disrupt sleep patterns.

Exercise in appropriate amounts may improve sleep/wake cycles.[8] Excessive exercise, however, may not be beneficial. Also, exercise that is done in the evening hours or shortly before bedtime may actually have a negative impact on sleep patterns. Warm baths or showers before bed can also improve sleep. The bed should be used only for sleep, and such things as reading or relaxing during the day on the bed should be avoided.

Physicians may find that persons with brain injury will try over-the-counter sleep agents that contain dyphenhydramine. Dyphenhydramine has a strong anticholinergic property and may have a negative impact on cognition. In addition, many over-the-counter medications may interfere with the drug levels of other medications. Educating persons with brain injury and their families regarding the use of over-the-counter sleep aids may be necessary, as many see over-the-counter agents as relatively benign.

Once physicians determine that a sleep medication is necessary, there are many agents from which to choose. In general, sedating agents depress cognition, while stimulants heighten arousal. However, the response to hypnotics can be quite variable. Even though treatment needs to be individualized, there are some basic rules that are helpful to follow.

In general, physicians may want to avoid initial trials with a benzodiazepine. Although this class of medication is commonly used in psychiatry, demonstrating good safety and efficacy, it can be problematic when used to treat persons with brain injury. Benzodiazepines can impair cognition and thereby exacerbate behavioral dyscontrol. These agents are quick and reliable and may be necessary in emergent situations, but their effectiveness is likely due to general depression of arousal. Also, many persons using benzodiazepines have a difficult time the following morning due to a "hangover effect" that can be associated with these medications. If the physician does try prescribing a benzodiazepine, it is important to use one with an appropriate half-life. If an individual is having difficulty with sleep initiation, an agent with a relatively short half-life might be beneficial. If the individual is having difficulty with early-morning waking or frequent waking during the night, a longer-acting sleep aid may be indicated.

Trazodone may be an effective sleep agent for physicians to consider. This agent has a very low anticholinergic component and is an effective sleep aid. Typically this medication does not negatively impact cognition, and most persons with brain injury do not complain of the "hangover effect." If prescribing trazodone, as well as other psychotropic medications, physicians need to be wary of the potential danger of priapism, an uncommon side effect resulting in a persistent erection which is a medical emergency. This occurs in about 1 in 1,000 to 10,000 people.[9]

Some of the newer hypnotic agents such as zolpidem and zaleplon claim few negative cognitive effects. These medications have been on the market for relatively short periods of time, and data in this population are still pending.[10]

As with other aspects of medication management of persons with brain injury, it is possible that the current medication regime may be contributing to insomnia. Medications used for other aspects of the patient's care can contribute to this difficulty.[11] It may be appropriate to change the dosing schedule of these medications or to try medically appropriate alternative medications.

Finally, many persons with brain injury, especially early, need medications to improve arousal during the day as well as medications to help them sleep at night. Persons coming out of coma, for example, may find benefit with daytime stimulants. Stimulants have been used in treatment for patients with brain injury for many years.[12] There is some evidence that they may decrease impulsivity and enhance cognitive performance following traumatic brain injury and may be helpful early in the recovery.[13] Correction of the sleep/wake cycle using sleep aids in the evening and night hours and stimulants during the day hours shows some benefit in cognitive improvement and can enhance the initial response of persons with brain injury to neuropsychosocial treatment plans.

Mood instability

Variability in mood is common following brain injury. Mood can range from profound depression to euphoria, but it is also common for mood to range from some level of depression to irritability and anger. Variability in mood is frequently seen early during evolution from coma, and often is correlated with an underlying delirium. However, many persons with brain injury continue to have instability in mood later in their recovery course, after medical stabilization.

Mood instability is not a diagnosis, but rather a description of symptomatology. Physicians should again attempt to discern the etiology of the presentation, exploring multiple possible etiologies. Early in the recovery phase, underlying confusion or delirium must be considered, and appropriate medical consultation may be warranted. Once the person with brain injury is medically stable, physicians should take into account physical discomfort or pain, insomnia, fatigue, or even underlying mood disorder or psychosis as sources of mood instability. Addressing the phenomenology of the behavior will aid in medication choice. Once other causes of mood instability have been ruled out, physicians may need to address the labile mood with a trial of a mood-stabilizing agent.

Instability in mood may also be a result of a current medication. Physicians should examine the medication list and consider this possibility. For example, benzodiazepines can cause disinhibition leading to extreme mood swings and behavioral dyscontrol. This side effect can be misidentified as a primary mood instability. In addition, antidepressants may have the potential to induce mania or hypomania. Physicians may use psychostimulants to improve focusing and concentration, but these medications have the potential to activate, overexcite, and agitate persons with brain injury. The resulting behaviors can present as mood instability. If persons with brain injury are receiving psychostimulants and appear to be agitated, it may be beneficial to obtain objective data from therapists while physicians attempt trials with alternating dosages, dose times, and periods off that type of medication.

If physicians consider the addition of a medication at this point, mood stabilizing agents may offer relief. Anticonvulsants such as valproic acid and carbamazepine may be beneficial. These may be especially desirable if there is a comorbid seizure disorder. Actually, many persons with brain injury have a comorbid seizure disorder that is being treated with anti-epileptic medications such as phenytoin and phenobarbital. These medications have a fairly high incidence of inducing cognitive impairment, and using them for persons with brain injury may be less desirable than with the general population. In contrast, valproic acid and carbamazepine may offer appropriate seizure prophylaxis as well as provide mood stabilizing properties. Physicians may be able to work with neurologists in selecting a single agent that may address the need for seizure prophylaxis as well as offering mood stabilizing properties. Because of side effects including gastrointestinal (GI) upset, abnormal liver function, and blood dyscrasias that may complicate treatment with these medications, physicians need to obtain periodic lab work.

Lithium carbonate is also used in persons with traumatic brain injury and mood instability.[14] As with the general psychiatric population, this medication is less helpful in treating the depressive aspect of mood swings than mood elevation or intense irritability. A relatively narrow therapeutic range, associated tremor, and possible confusion may make the use of lithium undesirable in some persons with brain injuries. More recently, gabapentin and lamotrigine have been suggested as agents that may be useful,[15,16] but data on these agents as mood stabilizing agents in patients with traumatic brain injury are lacking at this time.

Finally, substance use and abuse, common among persons with brain injury, can also be the source of variable moods. Physicians who suspect substance use may need laboratory evidence to confront persons denying such activity or may need to seek information from collateral sources.

Depression

Physicians will often observe depression in persons with brain injury. It is frequently a result of the organic insult to the brain. Although poorly understood, trauma may have both short-term and long-term effects on neurochemicals and the body's response to them. In addition to being a result of physical, organic damage, depression is also commonly related to the extreme psychosocial stress associated with the change in lifestyle following brain injury. Even in persons with brain injury who seem to have very little awareness of their deficits, depression may be a significant problem. Symptoms may include anhedonia, lack of motivation, insomnia, hopelessness, worthlessness, and suicidal ideation, paralleling depressive symptoms in the general population. Survivor's guilt is common, as well as an extreme sense of loss as persons with brain injury perceive that they are no longer the people they used to be.

Following brain injury, however, depression may present as atypical and dissimilar to depression in the general population. Persons with brain injury may present as agitated, irritable, and combative, with significant behavioral dyscontrol. It is not uncommon for severely depressed persons with brain injury to present as if they had profound anxiety disorders, obsessive and compulsive disorders, or even psychosis. Poor cognition, denial, and difficulty in communication can make diagnosis of an atypical presentation of depression quite difficult.

The use of antidepressant medication in persons with brain injury can have a significantly positive impact on the their mood and ability to function, and may improve behavioral dyscontrol. Depressive episodes can worsen cognitive deficits, and antidepressant medications may be of benefit for helping both sets of symptoms. Depressive episodes can occur for months or even years, and it is extremely important to identify this potentially reversible cause of cognitive inhibition and possible decline.

Physicians should plan early for trials of antidepressant medications for those persons with brain injury for whom they are considering a diagnosis of depression. Their efficacy and comparatively safe side-effect profile may make them relatively desirable agents. In persons where depression may be in the differential diagnoses for the etiology of the behavioral dyscontrol and aggression, physicians may want to consider an initial trial of an antidepressant prior to embarking on a medical trial with a potentially more toxic medication.

There are multiple types and classes of antidepressant medication. Various studies suggest that the efficacy of all types of antidepressants may be somewhat similar.[17] Very few controlled studies have been done for use of these medications, however, in persons with brain injury.[18] When choosing a medication, physicians should prescribe medications with a lower potential for undesirable side effects. As in treating depression in the general population, the choice of medication may be driven by concern about a particular potential side effect for an individual. The clinician should consider the medication's affinity to a particular receptor site in anticipating potential side effects. For example, medications with an affinity for the histaminic receptors will more likely be associated with sedation, weight gain, and hypotension, while medications acting at dopaminic receptors will more often be associated with extrapyramidal side effects and elevated prolactin. Medications with an affinity to the cholinergic system may more likely be associated with blurred vision, dry mouth, memory impairment, and constipation. Antidepressants which are more alpha-adrogenergic may have a tendency to be related to postural hypotension, dizziness, and tachycardia.

Tricyclic antidepressants may have a greater impact on the cholinergic system than many of the newer agents. In addition, use of tricyclics for persons with brain injury may be undesirable due to the impulsivity commonly seen with traumatic brain injury. The potential for harm due to difficulties with impulsivity or cognitive impairment leading to an inadvertent overdose should be taken into account. Finally, the tricyclic class of medication can be dangerous in persons who are abusing alcohol or other substances. For these reasons, physicians should be wary when prescribing tricyclic antidepressants. A low-dose tricyclic medication may be useful at times for persons experiencing chronic pain. General practitioners and pain clinics frequently use low-dose tricyclic medication for that purpose.

Selective serotonin reuptake inhibitors (SSRIs) and dual serotonin and norepinephrine reuptake inhibitors can be beneficial in treating depression in persons with brain injury. These medications typically have low anticholinergic activity, fairly low sedation, and fairly low risk of orthostatic hypotension. Unfortunately, these medications can be associated with possible sexual dysfunction, GI effects, and possibly insomnia. For this reason, physicians should dose and monitor these medications appropriately. Physicians can often ameliorate the side effects through changing the dosage or dosage schedule of these medications. Moreover, an individual's willingness to accept temporary or even longer-term side effects may greatly improve with appropriate education and information. Finally, persons with brain injury may have a higher incidence of adverse side effects with psychotropic medications than the general population.[19]

Psychosis

Psychosis in cognitively impaired persons with brain injury may be difficult to diagnose. As a result, both under- and over-diagnosis of psychosis is common. To begin with, communication difficulties may lead to an inadequate description of the experience by persons with brain injury. Furthermore, misinterpretation by therapists due to aphasia may be problematic. Finally, physicians and therapists may misdiagnose confabulation as psychosis. However, psychotic symptoms can occur following brain injury. This is especially true early during the course of recovery (for example, ICU delirium is commonly associated with psychosis), but can occur at other times as well.

As discussed previously, physicians should explore the possibility that the psychosis is related to an underlying mood disorder. As in the general psychiatric population, severe depression or an underlying mania can be associated with psychosis in persons with brain injury. Use of medication for the psychosis may be warranted in addition to treating the underlying mood disorder in persons with brain injury who show both sets of symptoms. Aggressive treatment of the mood disorder may assist in eliminating the need for higher doses of long-term antipsychotic medication. In some persons with brain injury, a complete taper off of all antipsychotic medication may be possible.

In the past, physicians often used neuroleptics as their first-line choice for treatment of aggression in persons with brain injury. Experience, though, has shown that neuroleptics should be considered early if persons with brain injury are experiencing psychosis as the source of their aggression, but other less toxic medications may be considered in aggression absent psychosis. Clearly, many persons with brain injury who experience auditory or visual hallucinations or delusional thinking can benefit from a trial of neuroleptic medication. However, persons with brain injury often exhibit cognitive deficits, difficulty with communication, or confabulation that may be erroneously interpreted as psychotic symptoms. In these persons with brain injury, the use of neuroleptic medication may be problematic due to the risks of possible side effects. Even those persons with brain injury who have true underlying psychosis driving their aggression may benefit from lower doses of neuroleptic medication than typically used in the general psychiatric population. It is important to keep in mind that the anticholinergic effect of these medications can contribute to difficulties with cognition and may actually worsen the behaviors that persons with brain injury exhibit.

Neuroleptic medications carry unique side-effect risks that are less likely to occur with other psychotropic medications. Tardive dyskinesia is a risk associated with all neuroleptic medications, although there appears to be a higher risk with the older, traditional neuroleptics than with the newer compounds.[20] Tardive dyskinesia is characterized by involuntary choreiform, athetoid, or rhythmic movements. These can occur in multiple muscle groups but are most common in the tongue, jaw, or extremities. These involuntary movements can be quite debilitating and may be permanent and irreversible in some patients.[21] For this reason, close monitoring for any signs of tardive dyskinesia is important, using, for example, tracking devices such as the DISCUS (Dyskinesia Identification System Condensed User Scale) examination. The DISCUS is a psychometrically developed test that attempts to objectively identify and quantify abnormal movements in various muscle groups.[22] Many states mandate such side effect tracking when using neuroleptics in particular patient populations. Other less severe neuroleptic-induced dystonias are also possible, and may involve abnormal postures or muscle spasms that can develop with use of these medications. If muscles of the swallow reflex or breathing are involved, a life-threatening condition can result. Typically, the signs or symptoms of these problems develop within the first 7 days of starting or increasing the medication dosage.

Neuroleptic malignant syndrome is also a risk with the use of neuroleptic medication. In this syndrome, an individual may develop severe muscle rigidity and elevated temperatures. As stated in DSM-IV, it is accompanied by "two (or more) of the following symptoms: including diaphoresis, dysphagia, tremor, incontinence, and changes in level of consciousness raising from confusion to coma, mutism, tachycardia, elevated or labile blood pressure, leukocytosis, and laboratory evidence of muscle injury..."[23] The symptoms can vary, but often there is laboratory evidence of muscle injury, such as an elevated creatine phosphokinase (CPK). This disorder represents a medical emergency and may need treatment in an ICU. The estimated prevalence of this condition appears to be 0.02 to 3.23% in psychiatric inpatients receiving neuroleptic medications.[24] It occurs more frequently in males and in young adults, and may be more common in individuals with brain injury.[25] It also appears that this condition occurs more frequently with high-potency neuroleptic medication. Thus, it is imperative for appropriate, informed decision making to take place before beginning treatment with this medication, and consent of the person with brain injury (if competent for such decision-making) or their conservator (if they are not competent) must be obtained. Moreover, providing education and information regarding this condition to persons with brain injury, their family, and therapists is an important tool in monitoring for this potential side effect.

Neuroleptic-induced akathisia is also common in persons with brain injury being treated with a neuroleptic medication, who make subjective complaints of restlessness.[26] Frequently, persons with brain injury engage in fidgety movements such as swinging their legs or bouncing their feet while seated, pacing, or rocking from foot to foot. It often is a very uncomfortable feeling, and persons with brain injury may be unable to sit or stand still for even a couple of minutes. In very severe cases, they may be unable to maintain a position for more than a few seconds. These persons often complain of a sense of inner restlessness, most often in the legs, and of a compulsion to move their legs with distress if not allowed to do so. These symptoms typically occur within 4 weeks of initiating or increasing the dose of neuroleptic medication. Treatment for this condition may involve a change or reduction in neuroleptic medication, or the use of medication such as anticholinergic agents to treat acute extrapyramidal side effects. It is fairly common for persons with brain injury who experience acute akathisia to engage in aggressive or violent behavior. For this reason, acute akathisia should be considered as a source of aggression in persons with brain injury who are treated with a neuroleptic medication.

Use of neuroleptic medication may also be associated with a postural tremor in persons with brain injury who have a pre-existing tremor related to their brain injury or have gait or balance disturbances. This may be especially problematic, and physicians should monitor this as well. Consideration should be given to reexamination of the current medication regime or a referral to a neurologist knowledgeable in treating tremor disorders.

Neuroleptic-induced parkinsonism also can occur with use of neuroleptic medication. The signs and symptoms related to this condition include tremor, muscle rigidity, or akathisia that often parallels the presentation of a patient with Parkinson's disease.[27] Again, these symptoms typically develop with use of neuroleptic medication either with initiation of the medication or with an increase in the dose of the medication. Close monitoring of persons with brain injury for this condition and the possibility of a decrease in neuroleptic exposure or use of an anticholinergic agent should be considered. Again, physicians should be wary of the potential negative cognitive impact of the use of anticholinergic medication.

As with antidepressant medications, the potential for particular side effects often drives the selection of a specific antipsychotic. In general, many of the newer or "atypical" antipsychotic medications seem to have a cleaner side-effect profile, and as a general rule may be preferable to the older, traditional antipsychotic medications. However, some of the older antipsychotic medications may be somewhat more sedating than the newer ones, and that aspect may be preferable for some persons with brain injury, at least temporarily. The goal should be to avoid anticholinergic effects, if possible, as well as orthostatic hypotension in persons who may be sensitive to this condition or who may be at higher risk for falls.

Anxiety

Anxiety is common following brain injury. Adjustment issues and grief of loss may evoke significant anxiety. Although anxiety may be temporary, it is often a chronic problem. It frequently leads to social isolation and depression. It may negatively affect cognition, impair judgment, increase impulsivity, and trigger aggression.

Anxiety is often due to medication side effects. Prior to treating persons with brain injury with an anxiolytic agent, physicians should review their current medication regime to determine whether other medications may be a contributing factor for anxiety. Stimulants can cause or worsen anxiety.[28] Anxiety-like symptoms can also result from medications; for example, akathisia from neuroleptic exposure or other psychotropic medications.

As in the general psychiatric population, anxiety in persons with brain injury may represent a diagnosis in itself, on one hand, or may be merely a symptom of a separate psychiatric diagnosis, on the other. For example, anxiety may represent a symptom of an underlying major depressive disorder. Ultimate treatment of the major depressive disorder may eliminate the anxiety. It is also fairly common for persons with brain injury experiencing psychosis to have anxiety as a component of that illness. Successful treatment and elimination of the psychotic symptoms may alleviate their anxiety.

Environment can greatly influence anxiety. Awareness of the link between environment and anxiety offers physicians the opportunity to follow the neuropsychosocial approach for controlling and eliminating the anxiety. In addition to medication management, the neuropsychosocial approach may effectively treat symptoms of anxiety in persons with brain injury, especially if cognitive impairment is contributing to the anxiety.

If treatment warrants use of an anxiolytic, physicians may find an SSRI or a dual-acting antidepressant preferable to a benzodiazepine. As previously stated, benzodiazepines, quick and reliable, likely work by overall depression of the arousal system. They are quite useful in emergencies and are relatively safe when used appropriately. However, benzodiazepines can be associated with cognitive impairment; they can cause unsteady gait and slurred speech. Disinhibition is not uncommon with the use of these medications, making aggressive outbursts potentially more likely. In comparison, SSRIs tend to have a cleaner side-effect profile. There is, unfortunately, a delayed onset of action for the anxiolytic effect of an SSRI or dual-action agent, and physicians may choose a benzodiazepine temporarily as a bridge until anxiolytic effects from the SSRI or dual-acting agent occur. Buspirone, another option, is a non-benzodiazepine anxiolytic that purports to cause less sedation and less psychomotor retardation than its cousin, the benzodiazepine. Again, there is relatively little information on the use of this medication in persons with brain injury. It appears to be a fairly safe agent when used appropriately, but the data are still pending.

Beta blockers, used for years as antihypertensive agents, have also been used in general psychiatry for anxiety disorders, including anxiety disorders associated with phobias and panic attacks, and have been used with some success to treat aggression in persons with traumatic brain injury.[29]

The use of dopaminergic agents, such as L-dopa, has reportedly helped with explosive behavior, as well as with cognition.[30,31] The data are still lacking on these agents, but physicians could consider a trial of this type of agent. These dopaminergic agents seem to help with arousal and cognition, especially early in the recovery course.

Again, because anxiety can be so greatly influenced by environment, as persons with brain injury become more stable in their environment, more accustomed to a group home and their schedules for instance, physicians may be able to taper them down or off anxiolytics over a period of time.

Cognitive deficits

Behavioral dyscontrol may be a result of cognitive deficits. Difficulties with memory, perception, and interpretation of subtle social nuances often lead to behavioral dyscontrol, including aggression. Persons with brain injury often become suspicious or exhibit paranoia due to their faulty recollection and accounting of events or their misperceptions about the world around them, different from the perceptions held by others. Chapter 2 reviewed in detail the link between cognitive deficits and behavioral dyscontrol, and Chapter 3 discussed paranoia and its link with cognitive deficits.

Cognitive deficits following brain injury should not be progressive. Slight and transient declines in cognition may occur with fatigue or due to medication effect. If, however, a person with brain injury is experiencing a significant or progressive cognitive decline, physicians must consider a medical cause. Especially in the early months following brain injury, physicians must be aware of hydrocephalus, rebleed, or seizure activity and may need consultation with neurology or neurosurgery.

Many medications impair cognition and may be the source for the cognitive decline of a person with brain injury. For example, medication used for pain control or spasticity may result in cognitive impairment. It is important to address this possibility through consultation with the specific prescribing physicians. Furthermore, as noted previously, anticholinergic agents and agents with anticholinergic effects, medications often prescribed by collateral treating physicians or which are obtained over the counter, are often the source of cognitive impairment. Persons with cognitive deficits due to brain injury are highly sensitive to even minor side effects from medication. Therefore, even medications that traditionally have had a relatively benign side-effect profile can be problematic for persons with brain injury. For this reason, physicians must follow the medication regimes of persons with brain injury closely, updating them so that they can maintain appropriate oversight, and it is essential that therapists and family members call in all medication changes to their physician to facilitate this process.

In contrast, unfortunately, there are very few medications that lead to cognitive improvement in persons with brain injury. If they do experience cognitive improvement, it is most likely a result of cleaning up the medication regime, diagnosis and treatment of an underlying medical condition, or treatment of a psychiatric illness such as a superimposed depression or psychotic disorder. However, physicians may find success in addressing difficulties with arousal through medication. Arousal is the gate-keeping mechanism through which the brain derives other cognitive activities. Difficulties with arousal can have a profoundly negative impact on attention, concentration, memory, and other higher-level cognitive functions. For this reason, close attention to the arousal of persons with brain injury becomes important.

Medications which improve arousal can have a positive impact on attention, concentration, and focusing, which in turn may improve the overall cognitive functioning of persons with brain injury and their ability to function in the real world. Psychostimulants seem to have a beneficial effect on cognition, even in persons absent an obvious mood disorder. Psychostimulants may improve the overall recovery curve following brain injury and do not appear to have a significantly detrimental impact on seizure threshold.[32] The use of psychostimulants does, however, have the potential for increased agitation and physical aggression. It is difficult to determine prior to treatment which persons will respond favorably to a psychostimulant. Therefore, the inability of persons with brain injury to concentrate, focus, and attend to task may warrant a trial of a psychostimulant. Educating them and their families about psychostimulants may alleviate the reluctance they may express regarding a trial of a psychostimulant. L-dopa has also been shown to have a positive impact on arousal and may be beneficial in promoting improved cognition, especially early during cognitive recovery.[33] SSRIs and dual-action re-uptake inhibitors may have a positive impact on cognition independent of the antidepressant and anxiolytic effects of these medications. Physicians now consider the use of these medications in persons with attention deficit disorder with evidence of some positive cognitive effects.[34,35] Therefore, physicians may want to examine the potential for using these medications for persons with brain injury.

Medications used for progressive dementias (e.g., donepezil, rivastigmine, and tacrine) have not yet been proven to have efficacy in persons with brain injury, although trial data are pending at this time.[36]

Sexually aggressive behavior

When persons with brain injury manifest aggression through sexually inappropriate or sexually aggressive behavior, physicians must consider the underlying cause of the aggression. Disinhibition, which is common with frontal-lobe injury, can lead to sexually inappropriate behavior. If such behavior is due to disinhibition, it commonly results in other inappropriate behaviors beyond those that are sexually inappropriate. How to address such disinhibition is found earlier in this chapter. Also, persons with brain injury who have secondary mania related to brain injury may have sexually inappropriate behavior as a component of their presentation. Because this symptomatology typically contains other inappropriate behaviors, physicians ought to consider the possibility of adding or increasing a mood-stabilizing agent as part of the medication regime.

Sexual aggression, however, can be in itself a target symptom following brain injury. The pathophysiology behind such a presentation is unclear, but sexually aggressive persons with brain injury can be extremely dangerous. Hormonal treatments may be appropriate. Medroxyprogesterone acetate is a progestin which can be given in injectable form and can be useful in persons with persistent hypersexuality often associated with aggression.[37] Progestins carry unique side effects, however. Males treated with progestins may develop secondary feminizing effects. Physicians must obtain proper informed consent, as discussed earlier in this chapter, before a trial of a hormonal treatment.

Conclusion

Medication management in persons with traumatic brain injury requires a thoughtful and systematic approach. Difficulties often arise due to their unique presentations, unpredictable responses to standard treatment regimes, and compliance issues. Improvement in treatment success occurs with input from a supradisciplinary team while developing, testing, and redefining the treatment hypotheses. More research and data are greatly needed in the treatment of this patient population, but the approach described here for medication management should allow the physician to develop treatment plans for improved target symptom control while improving the patient's independence and quality of life.

References

1. Johnson, R. and Balleny, H., Behaviour problems after brain injury: incidence and need for treatment, *Clinical Rehabilitation*, 10, 173, 1996.

2. American Psychiatric Association Staff, *Diagnostic and Statistical Manual of Mental Disorders*, 4th ed., American Medical Association, Washington, D.C., 1994, 146.
3. Giacino, J.T. and Cicerone, K.D., Varieties of deficit unawareness after traumatic brain injury, *J. Head Trauma Rehabil.*, 5, 1, 1998.
4. Temkin, N., et al., Valproate therapy for prevention of posttraumatic seizures: a randomized trial, *J. Neurology*, 91, 593, 1999.
5. Glenn, M., A Differential diagnostic approach to the pharmacological treatment of cognitive, behavioral, and affective disorders after traumatic brain injury, *J. Head Trauma Rehabil.*, 17, 273, 2002.
6. Lezak, M., Memory complaints that are not memory problems: identification, evaluation, and counseling, presented at 3rd Annual Managing Challenging Situations in Brain Injury Care, St. Paul, MN, September 27, 2002.
7. Garcia-Rill, E., Disorders of the reticular activating system, *Medical Hypotheses*, 49, 379, 1997.
8. Thaxton, L. and Myer, M., Sleep disturbances and their management in patients with brain injury, *J. Head Trauma Rehabil.*, 17, 335, 2002.
9. Banos J., Bosh, F., and Farre, M., Drug-induced priapism, its aetiology, incidence, and treatment, *Medical Toxicol. Adverse Drug Experience*, 4, 46, 1989.
10. Puzantian, T. and Stimmel, G., Review of psychotropic drugs, *CNS News Special Edition*, 3,13, 2002.
11. Eddy, M. and Walbroehl, G., Insomnia, *Am. Fam. Physician*, 59, 1911, 1999.
12. Lipper, S. and Tuchman, M., Treatment of chronic post-traumatic organic brain syndrome with dextroamphetamine: first reported case, *J. Nervous Mental Disease*, 162, 366, 1976.
13. Evans, R. and Gualtieri, C., Psychostimulant pharmacology in traumatic brain injury, *J. Head Trauma Rehabil.*, 2, 29, 1987.
14. Glenn, M.B., et al., Lithium carbonate for aggressive behavior or affective instability in ten brain injured patients, *Am. J. Phys. Med. Rehabil.*, 68, 221, 1989.
15. Fischer, J. and Patel, T., Guide to antieleptic agents 2001, *CNS News Special Edition*, 3, 101, 2001.
16. Leadbetter, R., et al., Mood-stabilizing properties of lamotrigine: a review of data from controlled clinical trials, *Psychiatr. Ann.*, 32, 766, 2002.
17. Geddes, J. and Butler, R., Depressive disorders, *Clinical Health*, 7, 74, 2002.
18. Busch, C.R. and Alpern, H.P., Depression after mild traumatic brain injury: a review of current research, *Neuropsychol. Rev.*, 8, 95, 1998.
19. Arciniegas, D., et al., Neuropsychiatric aspects of traumatic brain injury, *Curr. Treat. Options Neurology*, 2, 169, 2000.
20. Casey, D., Will the new antipsychotics bring hope of reducing the risk of developing extrapyramidal syndromes and tardive dyskinesia?, *Int. Clinical Psychopharmacol.*, 12, S19, 1997.
21. Barnes, T. and McPhillips, M., Novel antipsychotics, extrapyramidal side effects and tardive dyskinesia, *Int. Clinical Psychopharmacol.*, 13, S49, 1998.
22. Kalachnik, M., Ed., *Applied Tardive Dyskinesia Monitoring*, 2nd ed., Minnesota Department of Human Services, St. Paul, 1992.
23. American Psychiatric Association Staff, *Diagnostic and Statistical Manual of Mental Disorders*, 4th ed., American Medical Association, Washington, D.C., 1994, 739.
24. Lazarus, A., et al., The Neuroleptic Malignant Syndrome and Related Conditions, *American Psychiatric Press*, Washington, D.C., 1989.

25. Pelonero A., Leveson, J., and Pandurangi, A., Neuroleptic malignant syndrome: a review, *Psychiatric Services*, 49, 1163 1998.
26. American Psychiatric Association Staff, *Diagnostic and Statistical Manual of Mental Disorders*, 4th ed., American Medical Association, Washington, D.C., 1994, 744.
27. American Psychiatric Association Staff, *Diagnostic and Statistical Manual of Mental Disorders*, 4th ed., American Medical Association, Washington, D.C., 1994, 736.
28. Arciniegas, D., et al., Neuropsychiatric aspects of traumatic brain injury, *Curr. Treat. Options Neurology*, 2, 169, 2000.
29. Elliot, F., Propranolol for the control of belligerent behavior following acute brain damage, *Ann. Neurology*, 1, 489, 1977.
30. Fava, M., Psychopharmacologic treatment of pathologic aggression, *Psychiatric Clinics of North America*, 2, 427, 1997.
31. Smith, D. and Perry, P., Nonneuroleptic treatment of disruptive behavior in organic mental syndromes, *Ann. Pharmacotherapy*, 26, 1400, 1992.
32. Wroblewski, B., et al, Methylphenidate and seizure frequency in brain injured patients with seizure disorder, *J. Clin. Psychiatry*, 53, 86, 1992.
33. Fann, J. and Uomoto, J., Cognitive improvement with treatment of depression following mild brain injury, *Psychosomatics*, 42, 48, 2001.
34. Hedges, D., et al., An open trial of venlafaxine in adult patients with attention deficit hyperactivity disorder, *Psychopharmacol. Bull.*, 31,779, 1995.
35. Findling, R., et al., Venlafaxine in adults with attention-deficit/hyperactivity disorder: an open clinical trial, *J. Clin. Psychiatry*, 57, 184, 1996.
36. Blount, P., et al., Clinical use of cholinomimetic agents: a review, *J. Head Trauma Rehabil.*, 17, 314, 2002.
37. Britton, K., Medroxyprogesterone acetate for the treatment of aggressive hypersexual behavior in traumatic brain injury, *Brain Injury*, 104, 71, 1998.

chapter seven

Community placement using the neuropsychosocial approach

Introduction

Human beings strive for independence. The top two signs of independence in our culture are the capacity to drive a motor vehicle and the ability to live independently. Of the two, independent living is the harder to accomplish, evidenced by its typically being achieved by people notably later in the developmental progression from adolescence to adulthood. It is also the more important of the two for persons with brain injury with regard to their sense of self-esteem. That is, while it is devastating for persons with brain injury to be told that therapists are going to prohibit driving, it is terrifying for them to be informed that therapists will require group home placement, or worse, residence in a nursing home or state hospital.

To most persons with brain injury, living in a group home represents a failure in life. It is a direct affront to their identity as independent and self-sufficient members of society. In fact, most people in society are far less self-reliant than they think. Few people today can maintain their car without help. Those who can fix their car certainly cannot manufacture the parts or tools necessary to do so; furthermore, they are obviously incapable of producing the oil, antifreeze, and gasoline to make it perform. Few people can grow their own food. Farmers and others who know how to plant and raise food crops depend upon the fertilizer, equipment, and pesticides that other people make for them. Houses are built by a team effort and require specialists such as architects and experts in construction. Moreover, even those people who can build homes need equipment and energy (e.g., electricity, batteries, and fuel) that they lack the knowledge to generate independently. This list is infinite: we are a dependent people. While there may be the occasional person who does have the skills and knowledge to perform any one of these tasks, no one can do them all without help — certainly not while maintaining a standard of living that includes social and leisure time. We are inter-reliant; it is an illusion to think otherwise.

Yet, it is a comforting illusion. People base their self-esteem on this illusion. At best it is reassuring, but in times of stress it is harmful, for it sets a standard that is unachievable. The damage that can arise from the belief that one is fully self-sufficient becomes apparent when the most powerful sign of supposed independence — one's own separate residence, whether an apartment one pays for or a house one owns — is removed. Living in a congregate residence forces people to face their inter-reliance.

The challenge for persons with brain injury facing communal living is to recognize that where they live does not determine whether they are dependent or not. They can live in a communal setting and be inter-reliant, not dependent. Inter-reliance means that people assist each other's wellbeing. The opportunity to contribute to other people need not end because they live in a multiple-person residential setting. The key is to realize the ways in which, even when living in a group setting, persons with brain injury can find ways to benefit other people.

Even the most severely injured persons with brain injury can help other people to live better lives. Most importantly, they may serve as examples of how to cope under stress. Unfortunately, many people in society downplay the contribution of people who exhibit courage in the face of brain injury and only see their impairments and limitations. Society mistakenly thinks that *all* that severely injured persons with brain injury have to offer is their courage because they are unable to work or care for themselves. This attitude is extremely shortsighted. Society wants to pity those people with cognitive or physical limitations that interfere with self-care, driving, or work. However, practically everyone in society can do these things: they bestow no great distinction. In contrast, the ability to be a role model of perseverance and grace in the face of disability for other people is a special talent. Severely injured persons with brain injury who demonstrate compassion for others, persistence in striving for advancement, and courage offer other people examples of how to live. Persons with brain injury who serve other people as role models in exchange for assistance with activities of daily living or financial support give much more than they receive. It is important that persons with brain injury and those who know them understand that getting help with physical and cognitive concerns in exchange for providing insights into coping with life raises serious questions about exactly who is "reliant" on whom.

Recently, a person with brain injury died in a large city. He had faced a number of physical and cognitive impairments and had struggled over the years with work and living arrangements. He had always seemed to be in transition. He had exhibited behavioral problems, too, and sometimes had been physically aggressive. Nevertheless, the characteristic he was best known for was his optimism and his spirit. He was always talking about his most recent achievements and his goals. The tenor of his conversations was constantly one of hope, not lack of awareness. Furthermore, he was always glad to see whomever he was talking with; he always told people he talked to how much they meant to him; he always asked, with real interest and sincerity, about how other people were doing.

When he died, literally hundreds of people came to his funeral. It appeared that everyone who knew him came to the funeral. Their presence was a demonstration of the degree to which he had touched their lives. People were better people for having known him; therapists were better therapists for having known him. There are now thousands of people who receive better care because of the impact this one man had on persons with brain injury, their families, their therapists, and their government. He did not have this impact because of his job, his driving, his place of residence, or his "self-reliance."

A young, novice orderly once worked in a hospital where a young woman died due to organ failure after a prolonged hospitalization and much expensive care, with considerable distress to her family. To this orderly, the death seemed pointless and, if inevitable, ought to have at least happened quickly. There had to be meaning in how this woman died. Eventually, the orderly figured out that the meaning was the potential impact on others, himself included. That is, if he and others, but at least he if no one else, were different because of seeing her die — by learning new behaviors, having more compassion, by changing careers, anything — then he *created* meaning by knowing her. Despite all of her problems, and her eventual death, if he were different — and did not forget her — then she had made a contribution to society; she was inter-reliant, not dependent, even as she died, because he made her so.

Thus, it is important to realize that persons with brain injury living in communal settings are not dependent. Some persons with brain injury work, drive, are "self sufficient" in activities of daily living, and their "independence" is clear. Others are proactive role models of strength in the face of adversity, like the person with brain injury above who recently died. Still others are catalysts for other people to gain insight, and their lives may have an impact they will never know. Helping persons with brain injury complete activities of daily living in exchange for "just" having one's life changed is a fair trade. Living in a communal setting does not remove the opportunity to change other people's lives.

Finally, the idea of neuropsychosocial treatment becomes easier to grasp for persons with brain injury and their therapists when they both acknowledge that everyone is inter-reliant. As Condeluci noted, when people recognize that the locus of problems should shift from being inside the person to how the environment is structured, therapists can then attend to environmental change, rather than internal change.[1]

Availability

Despite the benefits of community living over institutionalization in nursing homes or state hospitals, many communities lack sufficient group homes with expertise in behavioral management after brain injury. This scarcity of congregate living sites is a function of three factors: a "not in my backyard" (NIMBY) mentality, flux in community philosophy regarding the nature of congregate living, and funding.

Not in my backyard (NIMBY)

The NIMBY problem is not unique to brain injury group homes, but it is more surprising when applied to group homes serving persons with brain injury than when applied to other types of group homes. Homeowners typically revolt against group homes in their residential areas because they choose to define the particular disability population as different from themselves. This is all too easy when they are certain that they *are* different from persons with a particular disability. They may have little interest in the needs of persons with mental retardation if their own children were born "healthy." Similarly, a mental illness that tends to first manifest itself when people are young may engender little sympathy among people whose perceived property values are at risk from a proposed group home if they are past the age of likely onset. However, while homeowners can fight to maintain property values over providing service for persons with disabilities that they no longer have to worry about personally, everyone is vulnerable to having a brain injury caused by a drunk driver. It is terribly short-sighted for people who resist having group homes for persons with brain injury in their neighborhood to ignore the risk that the very service they fight against may be needed for themselves or their family members, friends, or coworkers as soon as the very next automobile ride! Brain injury "does not discriminate."[2]

Community philosophy

Community philosophy regarding the design and nature of residential settings for persons with brain injury also determines group home availability. The growing zeitgeist in some locales is to discourage even four-person residential settings, as there is a push for more natural, home-based services or at least semi-independent living site service provisions. This trend follows past pushes from state hospital institutional placements into relatively large, but at least community based, settings (perhaps eight people or more in a building), and then a subsequent preference for the smaller sites of four-person group homes.

The trend to discourage even four-person group homes is commendable in the aggregate because many persons with brain injury can handle living arrangements that more closely approximate pre-onset living arrangements or that achieve even better community reintegration than do group homes. However, as applied to persons with brain injury who exhibit severe behavioral dyscontrol, it is troubling. Most persons with brain injury who continue to exhibit severe behavioral dyscontrol despite insight-oriented, contingency management, and skill-building therapies, need a neuropsychosocial approach to be successful. It is challenging enough in the first place to design neuropsychosocial environments that transfer from a program to a group home, but sometimes the challenges to devise ones that permit transfer directly from a program to settings even less structured than group homes can be insurmountable. Relatively unstructured, unsupervised home-based living presents many more opportunities for untrained community contacts to disrupt the neuropsychosocial behavioral management plan, leading to behavioral outbursts on the part of persons with brain injury and perhaps even hospitalization. On the other hand, persons with brain injury who benefit from a neuropsychosocial approach can eventually move from group homes into home-based or semi-independent living environments, but therapists very carefully plan such moves over time after experience monitoring them in community trials from the base of a group home. To move persons with brain injury from highly structured programming directly to unsupervised full community integration while maintaining their neuropsychosocial plan is fraught with opportunities to fail. Group homes are an excellent intermediary step, and in some cases a necessary permanent placement.

Funding

It is hard to develop the funding streams and provider networks necessary to ensure a sufficient amount of high quality residential sites for persons with brain injury. It is easier to articulate a theoretical position on group homes than it is to have bricks and mortar available as real homes with concrete services in place for this population. There is a risk that funding will be cut for current resources based on a philosophical belief about how ideal services should be offered, while only promising future funding, and even that with only questionable monetary support of a permanent secure nature. Persons with brain injury can lose current resources with just promises of a better world. Moreover, sometimes there is a lack of evidence that a newly proposed approach will work for the treatment of severe behavioral dyscontrol after acquired brain injury.

Sometimes the philosophy about what type of services lawmakers will support for persons with brain injury changes with shifts in the political winds, and as a result, persons with brain injury and therapists find their planning affected. Sadly, persons with brain injury and therapists whose efforts are being discussed typically have little authority over politicians and planning agencies who struggle over who will pay for services. While such battles take place behind the scenes, the vacuum in group home availability can be terrible, as therapists await assurances that there will be adequate development and program money.

Hence, the presence of funding also determines group home availability.[3] In part, providers develop group homes when there is sufficient money to run group homes. A challenge arises when funding resources allocate only enough money to manage typical group homes (i.e., group homes for persons with brain injury without behavioral dyscontrol problems), not those specializing in behavioral disturbances after brain injury. The costs are higher to serve persons with brain injury who demonstrate behavioral dyscontrol. Furthermore, even when enough funds exist to operate a group home for persons with brain injury who exhibit behavioral problems, there is often no money available prior to opening the doors to purchase the house and train therapists before the persons with brain injury arrive and service provision begins.

Funding is inextricably linked to payor source. Many health insurance companies exclude group home payments from their policies, arguing that "residential" costs are not "health" care costs, but rather are housing expenses. Our resource system is replete with examples of excluding coverage after injury or illness and cost shifting by dumping such expenses onto government-run insurance programs. Even many disability policies or long-term care insurance policies have restrictions that allow reimbursement sources to escape financial responsibility for group homes. In fact, many people buy an inadequate amount of disability and long term care insurance or have policies with limitations that will prove the policies to be insufficient, if the policy owners ever need them. This means that most people with brain injury will face funding dilemmas when they need group homes.

Implementation of the neuropsychosocial approach

Who group homes accept

Group home providers vary in their effectiveness in helping persons with brain injury who have behavioral dyscontrol. This is partly a function of whether or not their mission is to serve persons with behavioral dyscontrol. While many group home providers who lack expertise in behavioral dyscontrol after brain injury reject persons with behavioral dyscontrol, some group homes similarly lacking such expertise nonetheless accept them. They then do a poor job of providing services because they are unprepared for behavioral dyscontrol. To their credit, group home providers struggle under an unfair burden. They receive pressure from family members, referral sources, and funding sources to accept persons with brain injury who exhibit severe behavioral dyscontrol. At the same time, the available treatment models emphasize an inadequate traditional approach. However, when therapists do use environmentally based approaches, community success is obtainable.[4] Hence, it is crucial that group home providers know what it will take to handle behavioral dyscontrol, and make a decision to provide the necessary services to be effective.

The most crucial aspect of effective group home management of behavioral dyscontrol is construction of the correct neuropsychosocial environment. Disaster and crisis hospitalization await persons with brain injury if group home therapists fail to follow through with the neuropsychosocial behavioral management plan. If front line group home therapists do not understand, accept, and implement the appropriate neuropsychosocial environment, relapse of behavioral dyscontrol will occur.

Group homes must also consider other variables when deciding whom to accept. First, gender can be a concern. Most group homes are single-sex sites. However, group homes often give less consideration to the behavioral impact of the gender of therapists on group home residents than they do to matching the genders of the persons with brain injury who will live at a particular site. Some persons with brain injury do better with therapists of the same sex, and some do better with therapists of the opposite sex. Sometimes a mix of male and female therapists is better to handle different issues as they arise. Group homes should research the behavioral history of applicants for whether the gender of therapists makes a difference in each case. Sometimes it does not matter and sometimes it makes a great deal of difference for behavioral control. Obviously, group homes must follow legal hiring practices, but they should be aware of the effect of gender variables on behavioral dyscontrol.

Group homes should evaluate whether the physical attributes of an applicant are important for a particular site and group of therapists. The first of these attributes is the applicant's size. The same behavior may require a different neuropsychosocial approach when exhibited by a 6 foot 5 inch, 280-pound person rather than a 5 foot 7 inch 150-pound person. An applicant's strength is similarly worthy of consideration, because stronger individuals may pose a greater risk of harm to therapists when they demonstrate behavioral dyscontrol, and may require a different plan. The speed of movement and mobility of an applicant are additional variables for group homes to reflect upon. None of these variables, of course, contraindicates group home acceptance and management of persons with brain injury who exhibit behavioral dyscontrol. Tall, heavy, quick, mobile, and strong persons with brain injury can do well in group home settings, but group home therapists must know what variables they are able to handle.

Finally, group homes must know what supportive equipment, procedures, and medical complications they can manage. Equipment may include wheelchairs, walkers, braces, and canes. Procedures may entail communication through speech language typing/speaking devices. Medical complications vary greatly from individual to individual. Persons with brain injury may need help with catheterization. They may have to undergo frequent kidney dialysis or need help with diabetes management. They may need help with cancer treatments or face death and dying issues. The range of equipment, procedures, and medical issues is unlimited, and situations can change over time as these needs of persons with brain injury lessen, stabilize, or worsen. It can be heartbreaking for persons with brain injury who, after a period of behavioral dyscontrol, finally find that therapists at a group home have implemented the appropriate neuropsychosocial environment, making community placement realistic, but the opportunity is lost because the group home is unable to manage equipment, procedures, or medical needs. Hence, group homes must study not just their own neuropsychosocial capacity, but also the abilities of the group home therapists to manage complex medical issues.

Transition to group homes

There are unique issues regarding behavioral management during the period shortly after persons with brain injury arrive at group homes. The transitional period can present therapists with singular challenges. Persons with brain injury may present worse than their basal level. They may feel anger at being in the group home. They can be resentful and feel hurt because they were transferred to a congregate living site or to a different site from where they were living previously.

The challenge for therapists is to hold in abeyance first impressions which might have a long-lasting effect on their interactions with persons with brain injury. Awareness of the stress that persons with brain injury can experience during transition to a new living arrangement and its expression as behavioral dyscontrol can help therapists withhold premature judgment. Overreaction to early dyscontrol can be detrimental to long-term success. For example, therapists may decide that the neuropsychosocial behavior management plan is ineffective. As a result, therapists will sometimes resort to inappropriate punitive measures following episodes of behavioral dyscontrol. In some cases, therapists may feel that referral sources intentionally falsely described the persons with brain injury to gain their acceptance into group homes. Such suspicions interfere with consultations between group home therapists and referral therapists about how to implement neuropsychosocial plans. Finally, therapists must allow themselves sufficient time to become adept at implementing the neuropsychosocial plan. Behavioral control usually improves as therapists become skillful at creating the neuropsychosocial environment of new arrivals.

Conversely, there can be a honeymoon period when some persons with brain injury transition to group homes. For some, group homes represent a welcome alternative to state hospitals, jail, or locked nursing home units. Also, many persons with brain injury recognize the opportunity to create a good first impression in a new setting. In these cases, the trap that therapists must sidestep is that of assuming that early exemplary behavior is representative of baseline behavior. Only the passage of time will show whether persons with brain injury can maintain this behavior or whether they will regress to their normative level. Early on, therapists may feel a temptation to examine the neuropsychosocial plan and question its relevance in the face of ideal behavior. However, allowing for the honeymoon period to pass before shelving neuropsychosocial strategies will save therapists much anguish in the long run.

Advancement vs. stability

Therapists must strive for behavioral stability in the group home before considering expansion of the neuropsychosocial environment to additional settings. Too often, group home providers push for day program placement or vocational involvement shortly after persons with brain injury arrive. This can be a mistake. It is crucial to have a period of implementation of the current neuropsychosocial environment before attempting advancement to broader programming. It is easier to properly implement the neuropsychosocial environment in the group home, with group home therapists, than to try to do it correctly at the group home, on transportation, and at a day program or vocational site all at once. It is important to remember, persons with brain injury are not necessarily generalizing insight and skills to different settings, but rather that therapists in all these settings must be experts in how to act with persons with brain injury. Stability comes first, then expansion.

There may be financial pressures on group home providers to enroll persons with brain injury in day programs or vocation programs, regardless of whether it makes behavioral sense to do so. When persons with brain injury leave the group home during the day for off-site programming, the group home needs fewer therapists and therefore will incur less salary expense. Off-site programs may also tap funds from a different funding source than that which reimburses for group home expenses.

Nevertheless, unsuccessful behavioral plan implementation due to the failure of day program or vocational program therapists to conduct the correct neuropsychosocial environment also carries financial risks to the group home. Aggression can result in destruction of group home property that is expensive to fix or replace. It increases the risk of harm to therapists, in turn raising workers' compensation costs for the group home. It may lead to therapist turnover and associated costs of training new hires. Finally, it can lead to hospitalization of the aggressive person with brain injury, leaving an empty bed at the group home for which the group home loses reimbursement.

Persons with brain injury living in group homes are less likely to experience behavioral dyscontrol when the group homes provide services beyond just residential placement. When group home providers offer a broad range of services, they ensure that there will be consistent application of the appropriate neuropsychosocial environment. Therefore, some group homes provide their own off-site day programs. They act also as a transportation service. They may even provide therapists as job coaches. Such an integrated approach helps guarantee better coordination between support services, reduces the likelihood that an inexperienced therapist will contaminate the neuropsychosocial environment, and promotes better behavioral control on the part of the persons with brain injury who live at the group home. The persons with brain injury will encounter fewer situations and people that might trigger outbursts of anger when their residential, transportation, and day activity/vocational providers all know how to best help them maintain control.

Finally, from a system standpoint, behavioral stability should come before advancement. When there has been an expenditure of funds to develop an effective neuropsychosocial environment, it behooves therapists and payor sources to make sure that group homes successfully implement it before pushing for expansion to additional places and situations. Premature expansion, before therapists become astute at applying a neuropsychosocial plan, runs the risk of catastrophic failure and hospitalization. As already noted, group homes may mitigate some of the challenges of off-site programming by owning their own day program, vocational program, and transportation service. Still, for most persons with brain injury, group home therapists only offer traditional group home services, thereby necessitating that group homes ensure behavioral stability before allowing persons with brain injury to venture out to other environments.

Therapists

Roles

People are the most salient stimuli in anyone's world. For persons with brain injury living in group homes, the most important element for implementation of the neuropsychosocial environment is the group home therapists. It takes special therapists to understand their role in a neuropsychosocial environment, and the essential role that therapists play in creation of a neuropsychosocial environment in group homes cannot be overstated. In a group home when therapists fail to implement the correct neuropsychosocial environment, someone gets hit, behavior escalates, crisis ensues, and the person with brain injury ends up in the emergency room to be admitted to the hospital. Behavioral dyscontrol carries large risks with great penalties out in the community.

Expectations

Therapists must work hard to avoid the belief that it is unfair to treat everyone in a group home differently: some therapists believe they should treat everyone the same. The neuropsychosocial approach is based upon the belief that people should be treated according to their history and abilities, or more importantly, according to what works. What is effective is likely to be different for each person.

Therapists must be careful of the trap of thinking that the person with brain injury "should not do" something, "get away" with something, or "act that way." An alternative way to express the same idea is to say that the person with brain injury "should learn to do" something, "should act better," or "should conform." This is the familiar approach examined in a previous chapter that encompasses the belief that therapists ought to change the person with brain injury to fit in with society. Therapists may feel that there ought to be some consequence for the person with brain injury because of the behavioral dyscontrol (contingencies). At other times, therapists may believe that the person with brain injury ought to know better (insight). Finally, they may indicate that the person with brain injury should learn to act more appropriately (skill acquisition). Reverting to traditional conceptualizations of treatment is most common when therapists are frustrated by the behavior of persons with brain injury. However, it is destructive to return to such approaches if they have been shown to be ineffective for a particular person with brain injury.

Training

In order to create an effective residential program site, group home providers must train their therapists in the philosophy of the neuropsychosocial environment. Moreover, the therapists must accept that the group home's behavioral management approach depends upon their own behavior. Group home providers will find it easier to train therapists when their supervisors are experts in the neuropsychosocial approach to behavioral management after brain injury. The value of ongoing supervision and supervisor modeling of therapeutic behavior cannot be overstated. Modeling can lead to behavior and sociocultural change,[5] so it should be used by supervisors to influence the therapeutic approaches of the therapists.[6] Therapists should also attend workshops and seminars on behavioral treatment strategies, but these are inadequate without ongoing expert supervision. Therefore, both classroom instruction and appropriate supervision are essential for good application of a behavioral philosophy.

Knowledge about brain injury is essential for group home therapists to be successful. Unfortunately, it is all too common for group home therapists to have minimal, if any, formal training in brain injury. Efforts by the Brain Injury Association of America to certify therapists as having at least minimal knowledge in brain injury may help address this problem.[7] However, until this is in place, group home operators should provide training to their therapists to ensure the success of neuropsychosocial interventions and all other treatment approaches.

Group home therapists need to be educated about brain anatomy and physiology so that they are better able to appreciate why each individual's deficits lead to a different phenomenology of behavioral dyscontrol. Training must also include information about cognitive functioning. Therapists will do better when they are realistic about what persons with brain injury who exhibit behavior severe enough to require group home placement can understand and do. Study of neuropsychological reports and neuropsychosocial data will help therapists avoid being misled by self reports from persons with brain injury about their cognitive level of functioning and their reasons for their own behavior. It is just as unfair to expect persons with brain injury to perform beyond their abilities as it is to have unreasonably low expectations of them. Similarly, therapists must have training in how persons with brain injury present emotionally. Misreading emotional conditions can easily ruin the best neuropsychosocial plan, as many plans rely on therapists' responses to the emotional states of persons with brain injury.

Therapists who receive inadequate training in brain injury and behavioral dyscontrol can not only trigger dangerous behavior that can cause injury to themselves and their co-workers, but may set in motion serious physical and emotional consequences to persons with brain injury. Also, persons with brain injury may end up in a state hospital or jail if therapists do not understand brain injury and how to address behavioral dyscontrol. For these reasons, group home therapists must receive adequate training as an ongoing process.

Group home therapists who receive appropriate training typically demonstrate a dedication beyond that of many other providers to the needs of the persons with brain injury that they serve. The work of such group home therapists is frequently under-appreciated because they make their success appear so natural, but management of behavioral dyscontrol in a community setting is a very difficult task.

Previous experience

Group home providers for persons with brain injury often find it difficult to hire and keep good therapists. The market for good therapists is competitive, the work can be physically hard and emotionally draining, and the pay is less than ideal. Some group home providers for persons with brain injury hire therapists with experience in providing services to persons labeled "mentally retarded/developmentally disabled" (MR/DD). Many of these therapists struggle with the differences between those populations and persons with brain injury.

There are important differences between persons with brain injury and persons with mental retardation or developmental disabilities. It is important that therapists who are just beginning to work with persons with brain injury avoid the tendency to overestimate cognitive abilities based upon observation of cognitive strengths. Therapists with experience in developmental disabilities and mental retardation may miss the cognitive deficits of persons with brain injury. It is easy to misperceive the level of true judgment, problem solving, memory, and insight. Many persons with brain injury who have behavioral control problems initially present so well that therapists who lack brain injury experience misjudge how much structure they really require. Other differences between persons with brain injury and the MR/DD population are also important. Persons with brain injury who acquired their injury after a period of "normal" life have different expectations for themselves than do those with lifelong disabilities. Their benchmark for what they expect from themselves and how they anticipate others will treat them is founded on their life before onset. They often demand that other people deal with them as they were before onset, despite perhaps no longer having the cognitive, behavioral, or emotional skills they once possessed. Hence, therapists who come from a background of work with persons with mental retardation or developmental disabilities to provide care in a group home for persons with brain injury must make adjustments. They must re-conceptualize how they judge cognitive functioning and they must become adept at determining the degree of fit between the possibly overly high expectations of some persons with brain injury and their actual cognitive abilities.

Significant emotional trauma occurs around the changes brain injury imposes. Such changes induce guilt, anger, denial, etc., which have been explored in previous chapters. The presence of these strong emotions and the effect of brain injury on self-image require therapists to be aware of the importance of such factors for behavioral dyscontrol. Acquired brain injury imposes relatively rapid adjustment in comparison with the gradual awareness persons with mental retardation or developmental disabilities may experience as they mature and determine their strengths and limitations. This is not to say that living with mental retardation or developmental disabilities is easy or that this population avoids a sometimes painful acquisition of awareness of disability, but rather that each condition provides its own unique challenges. Therapists serving in group homes who have previously specialized in work with persons with mental retardation or developmental disabilities must adjust their perspectives to provide treatment for the emotional stresses experienced by persons with brain injury.

There is an additional difference between these fields. The goal of care for many group homes specializing in the needs of persons with mental retardation or developmental disabilities is usually to advance these individuals. Care plans are written in the language of progress, and the focus is on achievement of greater skills. The goal is to help persons with these difficulties obtain their maximum functioning. The belief in advancement as the purpose of care is part of a process that has been years in the making, and reflects a deep philosophical perspective held by the families of persons with mental retardation and developmental disabilities to help them overcome physical and cognitive limitations in the face of a safety net that tends to help only those people with strong family advocates who help them obtain resources. These advocates can look back over years of caring to see that never settling for being told that their loved one could not do something by poorly trained, uninformed, and uncaring "experts" has resulted in the achievements the person with disability can now claim.

A different scenario exists after acquired brain injury for persons who exhibit severe behavioral dyscontrol, and the goal of care must reflect this reality. Often persons with brain injury with severe behavioral dyscontrol have a problem that is the opposite of that of persons with mental retardation or developmental disabilities. Persons with brain injury who demonstrate behavioral dyscontrol often do so because the environment is too permissive. They fail behaviorally because there is little insight into the environmental structure they need in order to function well. Also, persons with brain injury arrive at their injury from a previous life of "independence," not having had to work hard for each achievement as persons with mental retardation or developmental disability might have done. Their history is not one of gradual advancement to obtain simple life successes, but rather one of "normal" development. Hence, after brain injury they expect a return to normal freedom. When they are unable to manage that freedom, behavioral dyscontrol ensues.

Therapists who have previously worked in group homes for persons with mental retardation or developmental disabilities must write treatment plans to better match with the needs of persons with brain injury who exhibit behavioral dyscontrol. Therapists should be aware of the differences between the needs of these populations to devise treatment plans for persons with brain injury who exhibit behavioral dyscontrol where the measure of success is first behavioral stability, not skill development, participation in various programs, or independent living. While such goals should be supported when feasible, therapists must account for the importance of the neuropsychosocial environment to avoid increased risk of behavioral regression and hospitalization.

A note of caution is warranted. Many persons with brain injury do in fact experience unfair limitations that society imposes upon them. Strong advocacy to help persons with brain injury fight against unreasonable and uninformed judgments against them should be encouraged. Persons with brain injury and their supporters have many battles still to fight so that they can achieve their maximum potential. Yet when it comes to severe behavioral dyscontrol, the problem is usually not that of too many restrictions (though sometimes this can be the case), but rather of poorly construed neuropsychosocial environments. Therapists and group home providers must appreciate this in order to be successful.

These differences account for why mixing persons with brain injury and persons with mental retardation or developmental disabilities together in group homes can fail. The goals of care and the expectations of the persons being served as well as the perspectives of knowledgeable therapists are too different. These differences are not merely ones of casual reflection, but are essential for therapists to appreciate if they are to achieve treatment success with persons with brain injury. When programs attempt to mix persons with brain injury and persons with mental retardation or developmental disabilities, persons with brain injury may refuse to participate, exhibiting empathy for persons from the other populations and concern for their needs but vehemently asserting that persons with brain injury have different needs.

Therapist turnover

Therapist turnover in group homes can be high. High turnover is devastating to the neuropsychosocial environment because new therapists may disrupt the environment. New therapists may begin interactions with persons with brain injury without having studied the neuropsychosocial behavioral management plan. Referring therapists who have sent a person with brain injury to a group home may get calls from the group home therapists warning that behaviors are escalating and inquiring about what has been helpful in the past. When this happens in the case of a person with brain injury who has successfully been at the group home for a period of time and suddenly begins to struggle with behavioral control, it may be due to a recent turnover in therapists. The presence of new therapists with less education, training, or familiarity with a particular neuropsychosocial behavioral management plan may be a crucial factor in the resumption of behavioral dyscontrol. There may be other contributing factors, but therapist turnover should be looked at before pursuing other causes. A referring therapist may also inquire about what the new therapists at the group home have tried, focusing on their contribution to the environment and whether the steps that have been undertaken are part of the neuropsychosocial plan. It is too easy for new therapists to fall back on preconceived notions about behaviors, expectations for how persons with brain injury "should" act, how they treat children, etc.

Therapists and boundaries

Therapists must exercise a certain degree of "rational detachment"[8] when working with persons with brain injury. Treatment should be based on cognitive, behavioral, and emotional data and the formulation of a neuropsychosocial environment. Persons with brain injury are not therapists' friends, children, spouses, or parents, and therapists must not let their behavior in other non-professional relationships influence treatment planning. It is unacceptable for therapists to base treatment techniques on what has worked for them in their non-professional relationships. (see Meehl.[9])

Therapists should pay diligent attention to their own behavior to heighten awareness of boundary issues. Violation of the professional boundaries between therapists and persons with brain injury is a concern in the provision of any treatment protocol. However, in neuropsychosocial treatment where there is such a strong emphasis on therapists' actions *as* the treatment itself, professional boundary violations are even more devastating to therapeutic success. Therapists must clearly understand their roles and should receive explicit training in the pitfalls of providing treatment in group home settings. Therapists should also be aware that adherence to boundary rules will protect them from accusations of inappropriate behavior and conflicts of interest.

Summary

Group home providers who specialize in services for persons with brain injury must be honest about their expectations when they hire therapists. They ought to be forthright about their standards for therapists in a neuropsychosocial treatment plan. Therapists should understand that the group home providers, as well advocates and families of persons with brain injury, will attend to therapists' behavior. Furthermore, therapists must receive sufficient training about brain injury and related issues. Providers who hire therapists without being clear about the importance of consistent, appropriate therapist behavior are setting the stage for chaos.

Physical space

An important component of the neuropsychosocial environment is physical space design. Group home therapists must carefully consider whether their sites are physically conducive to behavioral control. Although an infinite number of variables must be taken into account, a few factors can be particularly troublesome if improperly designed.

Most persons with brain injury do better behaviorally with private rooms. Previous chapters have already discussed issues related to privacy.

Obviously, having "housemates" is inherent in congregate living, but having "roommates" is frequently problematic. Friction leading to behavioral dyscontrol typically arises with roommates, because having a roommate often involves more intrusiveness than persons with brain injury who exhibit behavioral dyscontrol can tolerate.

A common area, such as a living room, is normally a part of a group home. However, a second common area, such as a finished basement, allows therapists to avoid behavioral escalation by being able to meet simultaneously with two groups of persons with brain injury in separate locations. Private bedrooms do not meet this need. They are frequently too small for multi-person activity and privacy or control issues will arise if therapists attempt to conduct activities with housemates in each others' rooms.

Therapists need a kitchen in which they can control availability of food, and kitchen implements and appliances. Depending upon the behavioral symptoms of the particular persons with brain injury residing at the site, they must be able to restrict access to food or to implements that persons with brain injury might use as weapons against themselves or others. Control of kitchen appliances may be necessary to ensure safety.

Bathroom availability can be a significant issue. Sufficient facilities must be present. Persons with brain injury who demonstrate behavioral dyscontrol tolerate delay in getting into the bathroom poorly. Housemates may unintentionally push this intolerance to the limit because of their own delays in leaving the bathroom due to impaired motor skills, slow processing speed, organizational difficulties, or perseverative/compulsive behavior.

One advantage of group homes over large congregate living facilities is often the availability of grassy yards that have personal touches and are inviting. It can be soothing to step outside. However, therapists may best utilize this space therapeutically when they can control access to it from the group home. In addition, a fenced-in yard will help prevent issues of aggression with neighbors, or elopement. Group home providers would do well to consider backyard features that include elements of therapeutic gardens. Such therapeutic spaces can help mitigate behavior.[10]

Family support

The value of family support for the neuropsychosocial environment in group home settings cannot be overstated. There is a greater potential for family members who act out of accord with the neuropsychosocial treatment plan to disrupt the care of persons with brain injury in these settings than there is in a more controlled setting such as a hospital. Hence, it is crucial that therapists and family members work together as a team in creating the neuropsychosocial environment.

When family members are supportive and realistic, they strengthen the effectiveness of the neuropsychosocial environment. Therapists can facilitate family input by including family wishes in planning and evaluation meetings. Family members who are dedicated to the treatment of persons with brain injury may travel hours to a group home to visit and reinforce the efforts of the therapists. Outings with family members can provide a source of pleasure for persons with brain injury as well as an opportunity to apply the neuropsychosocial environment outside of the group home.

Unfortunately, family members can also be detrimental to successful treatment. Sometimes family members are unaware of the impact of their attitude and behavior. There are many possible causes for this lack of awareness. Family members may be dealing with their own guilt about the life changes that brain injury has brought to their loved one. They may be unhappy about an element of the treatment program, and unintentionally communicate their dissatisfaction to the person with brain injury.

When problems caused by family members are unintentional and based on lack of awareness, therapists can help family members by providing them with education about brain injury, the neuropsychosocial treatment plan, and the effect of their behavior and attitude. In addition, it is important for therapists to incorporate family perspectives into treatment planning as family members adjust after they receive education. Finally, psychotherapy for family members may be helpful. Therapists often omit making referrals for psychotherapy for family members as persons with brain injury proceed through various stages of care. Group home providers may help families by recommending psychotherapy with a psychologist who has training in brain injury and family adjustment. After all, it is likely that the family is hurting, too. Many family members show symptoms of their own post-traumatic stress disorder as they respond to the trauma of seeing a loved one so badly injured.

In contrast to family members who are unaware of the problems they cause, some family members may intentionally undermine treatment efforts. Different family factions may fight over control of their loved one. They may argue about which family members will have guardianship or conservatorship of a person who is a minor with brain injury. Similar battles can occur over an adult. Some cases involve custody battles about the minor children of a person with brain injury. There are also family wars over the financial resources of the person with brain injury. Long-buried family wounds can reopen when family members who hold old resentments against each other must work together to benefit the person with brain injury. There can also be unresolved family differences about values that spill into treatment planning as family members fight out their value systems over the design of the care plan. Finally, there can be outright psychopathology among members of a family.

Therapists generally find that active sabotage of the care plan by family members is harder to address than unawareness that some family members may have about their impact on treatment. Active sabotage can range from family noncompliance to acting out hidden family agendas. Family members may try to split therapists. They may attempt to solicit one therapist to report on another. They may lie to therapists. Family members may even yell at therapists or threaten them with violence. Family members who undermine the neuropsychosocial environment can easily influence persons with brain injury. The lack of family support for implementation of the neuropsychosocial environment can easily ruin the best efforts of therapists.

Group home therapists must take action when family members exert a negative influence on the chances for persons with brain injury to succeed. Extreme behavior on the part of the family members requires strong therapist response. Therapists may need to limit family visits or, at minimum, supervise the visits. They may place restrictions on passes, requiring contact to take place on-site at the group home. Therapists may require an independent conservator be appointed as a prerequisite for continued care at the group home. When family behavior is truly detrimental to the welfare of a person with brain injury, therapists may have to make a vulnerable adult report to the authorities. Hopefully, therapists will rarely encounter family members whose behavior or attitude is harmful. Most family members are, in fact, active, dedicated participants in pursuing the best care possible, but therapists will occasionally encounter unacceptable family behavior.

Handling aggressive episodes

Introduction

It is essential that therapists who work with persons with brain injury who exhibit behavioral dyscontrol can maintain safety when episodes of aggression seem imminent. This applies in all settings, ranging from hospitals to group homes. Typically, however, there are experts in de-escalation techniques in hospital settings who are available to train therapists or assist during crises, while in group home settings therapists may have to fend for themselves. It is crucial that group home therapists know de-escalation processes and be behavioral experts themselves, although it is wise for group homes to have on-call supervisors and/or a crisis team. Of course, when therapists correctly design and implement the neuropsychosocial environment, there ought to be few instances of dyscontrol. Nevertheless, therapists may encounter situations that are unexpected, and preparation in handling episodes of aggression may mitigate the impact of aggressive episodes.

Preparation

Therapists need to know what the various guidelines permit them to do. They must adhere to federal and state rules, and training regarding this should be provided by hiring organizations. Therapists must also know their organization's policies and restrictions, including when their organization recommends that they call the police.

Therapists must be familiar with the responses of their teammates so they can account for the reactions of their co-therapists during a crisis. Therapists will be unable to contain episodes of behavioral dyscontrol when they cannot predict the behavior of other therapists during a crisis; if they are uncertain about the responses of their teammates, some therapist usually gets hurt. Teamwork helps avoid harm to therapists and to persons with brain injury.

Therapists should study the environment in which they work before an episode occurs. They must know how much space they have in which to maneuver, where equipment or furniture is commonly kept so that they do not trip on it, where the exits are and which doors are typically locked, which windows are breakable, etc. It is vital to appreciate what items in the environment persons with brain injury can make into weapons (e.g., the metal spine of a looseleaf binder, razors for shaving, glass from a picture frame, knives in a dishwasher). In fact, frequent periodic house searches may prove useful to locate and remove items that persons with brain injury may hide away. Therapists should look under rugs and mattresses, behind books on shelves, in the dirt of potted plants, etc. They should be sure that keys for group home vehicles are kept locked away and that their personal keys and purses are secure. Finally, therapists must be certain about the emotional and behavioral environment other therapists will create during a crisis.

In addition, therapists should be constantly alert regarding body position when dealing with persons with brain injury who have a history of aggression. They ought to avoid positions where persons with brain injury stand over them, such as when therapists are seated. They need to maintain appropriate spacing between themselves and persons with brain injury. When interpersonal space decreases, therapists should plan for how they might block a blow or a kick and position themselves accordingly.

Therapists should wear appropriate clothes when working with persons with brain injury, if they have a history of behavioral dyscontrol. An enraged person with brain injury can grab men's neckties or women's earrings; a necktie is a noose around the neck, and earrings can be ripped through the earlobe. Shoes should be flat, with closed toes. Open-toed shoes expose toes to damage, and high heels disturb balance. Long hair can make a tempting target for persons with brain injury to grab.

Intimate knowledge of the neuropsychosocial treatment plan and past history of behavioral dyscontrol is invaluable when therapists face potential episodes of behavioral dyscontrol. The decisions therapists make during a crisis ought to be based on knowledge of the functioning of the person with brain injury so that therapists' actions are not generic, but tailored to the individual responses of the person with brain injury. Therapists must continually monitor the emotional status of persons with brain injury who exhibit dyscontrol in order to enhance their own readiness for episodes of behavioral dyscontrol.

Episode management

Therapists' actions should have a clear purpose when dyscontrol occurs. The goal should be to deescalate the situation and to prevent injuries. Novice or less experienced therapists may lose sight of this goal during a crisis. They may fall into the trap of trying to enhance the insight of persons with brain injury while dyscontrol is occurring. They may attempt a therapeutic interaction. Worse, some therapists get caught up in trying to be right while arguing with distraught persons with brain injury who are threatening or engaging in aggression. Therapists who allow their egos to be challenged and try to win a power struggle often get physically hurt.

It is important to remain calm during crises involving aggression. Therapists must monitor and adjust their voice pitch and volume, facial expression, gestures, choice of words, speed of movement, and eye contact. Experienced therapists will consciously manipulate these variables to obtain their goal, particularly during behavioral crises. Therapists must remember that their natural responses as people may not be their best responses as therapists. They must not permit their natural emotional reactions (e.g., fear, anger, laughter, etc.) to dictate their responses, but must adjust their emotional armamentarium to control the situation. The goal is not to win during a crisis, but to deescalate the crisis without anyone getting hurt. All else is secondary, and other concerns can be addressed after the immediate crisis has passed.

Therapists who lack experience in behavioral dyscontrol after brain injury tend to make some predictable errors. It is common for them to get trapped by persons with brain injury into arguing about the facts of who did what that lead to the aggression. Novice therapists may then try to explain why the persons with brain injury showing dyscontrol were wrong in the situation. Such an approach is usually inflammatory. Similarly, therapists who provide explanations to persons with brain injury based on therapists' perceptions of the motive for aggression during crises are likely to worsen the situation. Also, therapists should avoid downplaying the reasons persons with brain injury give for their aggression. Saying they have no valid reason for aggression commonly leads to further aggression.

There are other mistakes that novice therapists can make. Generally, it is ill advised to threaten persons with brain injury with the consequences for their behavior when they are upset. Threats of punishment rarely deescalate crises and usually exacerbate them. Furthermore, some therapists may attempt to bluff about consequences, the actions that they will take, the resources they have available, etc. When persons with brain injury who are distressed fail to respond to the bluff and then realize that therapists were bluffing, they are less likely to trust the rest of the therapists' statements during the crisis. (Of course, this also destroys rapport for therapy later, and for interaction during the next crisis.) For the same reasons, therapists should also avoid promises of a positive nature that they cannot deliver to get persons with brain injury to calm during a crisis. Finally, therapists should avoid lying during crises. This, too, destroys credibility. It is easy for therapists to fall into the trap of saying whatever they think will placate persons with brain injury who are irritated, but this seeds the ground for further behavioral dyscontrol when the persons with brain injury detect the lie. Episodes of behavioral dyscontrol can be handled most effectively without bluffs or lies.

Therapists should avoid talking to each other to plot strategy while they ignore persons with brain injury who are having escalating behavior. If "sidebar" conversations are necessary, therapists should consult away from persons with brain injury during a crisis. Therapists who fail to direct their attention and conversation to the persons they serve during incidents of dyscontrol often inflame emotions and worsen behavior.

Despite the preceding cautionary notes, therapists can resolve behavioral dyscontrol events without anyone getting hurt. First, it is important to acknowledge the feelings of persons with brain injury when they are upset. It is a good idea to provide them time to vent their feelings; therapists should not rush to resolution of the incident if allowing expression of feelings leads to calmness. Periods of silence can be helpful. Many persons with brain injury need extra time to process when they are distressed. Sometimes therapists will determine that an offer to sit down and talk provides angry persons with brain injury needed attention while it also provides an out from a standoff. Providing choices, rather than directives, during a behavioral emergency is a helpful calming technique. If persons with brain injury issue challenges when angry, therapists will enhance the opportunity for success by ignoring the challenge. Discussion of the merits, nature, and likelihood of threats often disintegrates into unproductive debate, risking behavioral escalation. Moreover, as having an audience may exacerbate posturing for control, therapists will be more efficacious if they remove any unneeded bystanders.

The following phrases are helpful comments to take the conversation in a useful direction:

> Tell me what is happening.
> What can I do to help?
> You may have a reason to be upset. What should we do together?
> You may be right. Can we talk about this?
> This isn't working out very well. What else can we do?

These statements lead to dialog and a chance for persons with brain injury to relax and engage the therapists. They do not challenge or deceive, but solicit teamwork.

Crisis management requires a leader. For each crisis, it should be clear which therapist is in charge of the situation and will be making the executive decisions. This can be someone other than the most senior person on duty, and is usually either the therapist who has the most rapport with the person with brain injury or whichever therapist was present when the situation began, though in some instances the original therapist may be a trigger and helps best by leaving once another therapist takes charge. Obviously, the crisis leader must know how other therapists will respond during crises.

Environmental control is crucial during a crisis. Therapists should remove unnecessary bystanders. They should station themselves at entrances to control visitors from entering an area where a crisis is in progress. Also, therapists should know where exits are so they can evacuate quickly if the situation deteriorates. Other persons with brain injury should be directed away from the crisis.

All of these interventions entail multiple therapists. Thus, a team approach is essential. A team approach ensures that experienced therapists will avoid placing themselves in scenarios where behavior may deteriorate and only one therapist is present without backup. Therapists should always know how much backup they have, how to reach it, and how fast it will come. This includes police backup.

After any event, therapists should conduct a debriefing. Debriefings can increase therapists' sense of security. To conduct interactions with persons with brain injury who are distressed, therapists must feel secure. At the beginning of a debriefing, therapists should check to see if anyone was physically hurt, and if so, they should help obtain care for injured coworkers. Emotional debriefing is also wise. No therapist should feel that it is wrong to be afraid or upset. Team support is essential to make sure that everyone can decompress. Finally, therapists can make plans for how to avoid crises in the future and how to proceed better next time a crisis occurs. Crises are learning opportunities for therapists to refine the neuropsychosocial environment. Some of the most effective neuropsychosocial treatment plans arise from therapists' reflections about the antecedents of past crises. Examination of how therapists handle an episode of behavioral dyscontrol and which physical plant elements are a hindrance and which are assets leads to better preparation for any future occurrences.

Conclusion

Therapists providing treatment in group homes should take a great deal of pride in their work. They are helping persons with brain injury follow through on neuropsychosocial strategies that permit them to integrate back into the community to the maximum degree possible. Therapists working in group homes do this often with less support and resources than institutional therapists, in a setting with less structure and control, and often with more community and family pressure to advance those they help to a normal life. Despite these challenges, group home therapists frequently achieve remarkable success. Therapists who are successful in group home settings must come to terms with their own value system regarding independence, equality, and expectations for behavioral performance. They must receive training in brain injury in general and crisis management in particular. They must deal with boundary issues. The neuropsychosocial approach provides them with a methodology for their work in the challenging setting of group homes.

References

1 Condeluci, A., *Interdependence: The Route to Community,* 2nd ed., G.R. Press, Winter Park, FL, 1995, chap. 3.

2 Connors, S.H., *Resource Facilitation: A Consensus of Principles and Best Practices to Guide Program Development and Operation in Brain Injury,* Brain Injury Association of America, Alexandria, VA, 2001, 5.

3 *Returning to the Community: Persons with Brain Injury in Minnesota,* Minnesota Department of Human Services Community Supports for Minnesotans with Disabilities, St. Paul, 2000.

4. Feeney, T.J., et al., Community supports for individuals with challenging behavior after brain injury: an analysis of the New York State Behavioral Resource Project, *J. Head Trauma Rehab.,* 16, 61, 2001.

5. Bandura, A., *Principles of Behavior Modification,* Holt, Rinehart, and Winston, New York, 1969.

6. Wesolowski, M.D. and Zencius, A.H., *A Practical Guide to Head Injury Rehabilitation: A Focus on Postacute Residential Treatment,* Plenum Press, New York, 1994, chap. 5.

7. American Academy for the Certification of Brain Injury Specialists, *Guidelines for Certified Brain Injury Specialists,* Brain Injury Association of America, Alexandria, VA, 1998.

8. Hoffman, L., personal communication, 2002.

9. Meehl, P.E., Why I do not attend case conferences, in *Psychodiagnosis: Selected Papers,* P.E. Meehl, Ed., W.W. Norton, New York, chap. 13.

10. Wedel, A. and Giesschen, E., A growing perspective: interacting with nature to heal body and soul, presented at 17th Annual Brain Injury Association of Minnesota Conference, Brooklyn Center, May, 2002.

chapter eight

Clinical vignettes: demonstrations of the neuropsychosocial approach

Introduction

Imagine persons with brain injury being admitted to a program. Their records show they have done one or more of the following: assault their mother, burn down their group home, sexually assault someone, physically destroy a hospital nursing unit, assault police officers, try to kill their children, harass their physician's office personnel to the point of being banned from the physician's practice, run off with strangers for extended periods such that the police had to be called, abuse multiple illicit drugs and alcohol, steal property, attempt suicide numerous times, threaten to kill someone, etc. Now imagine a team of therapists reading such records and then responding with the sentiment that it is fortunate these persons with brain injury have come to their program! There is no sense of their being overwhelmed by these histories or of panic about what to do. In fact, the worse the behavioral history, the more these therapists want the case because they know they can make a difference. Persons with brain injury who exhibit the preceding behaviors are the kind of persons these therapists look forward to serving. These persons with brain injury need assistance, and these therapists know what to do: implement the neuropsychosocial approach.

Therapists who can apply the neuropsychosocial approach must have three sets of knowledge. First, they must grasp the basic information and theoretical perspective of the neuropsychosocial approach. This book provides that fundamental knowledge in Chapters 1 through 4. Next, therapists must have some typical, core procedures to follow to initiate care so that they can avoid reinventing the wheel at the start of every case. Chapter 5 provides this information. Finally, they must have a store of clinical experience to draw upon so that they can recognize similarities that exist between cases. This chapter will provide a start toward building a library of clinical experience and insights. The intent of this chapter is to bring to life the neuropsychosocial approach so that therapists can visualize examples of how they might proceed when they confront behavioral dyscontrol.

In truth, these are the three bodies of knowledge that any therapist in any field uses: basic information and theory, prepared procedures, and clinical experience. However, this chapter is not a compendium of interventions. Since each case of behavioral dyscontrol has case elements lacking in other cases, the neuropsychosocial intervention will be different for each person with brain injury. Therefore, there can be no comprehensive list of definitive interventions. Therapists must be innovative to be successful. This chapter is not a cookbook. There are no preset guaranteed recipes for achieving behavioral control. Even Chapter 5 makes the point that the behavioral plans it presents are initial plans, not final plans. Ultimately, therapists must devise a neuropsychosocial plan for each person.

This chapter presents vignettes that demonstrate what interventions look like. Therapists may never encounter a case that exactly fits one of these vignettes. This chapter should be used to see *how* experienced clinicians would *think* rather than exactly what they would *do*. This chapter will attempt to free therapists to think outside the box, or better still, to throw the box away.

Sometimes the neuropsychosocial approach involves a few "simple" changes, although these are usually based upon extended study on the part of therapists to gain insight into which "simple" changes to make. At other times, plans can be extraordinarily complex. Therapists should prepare to invest much time in developing neuropsychosocial plans. This may involve a lot of time finding "simple" solutions or a lot of time developing complex plans. Therapists should avoid being fooled into thinking that the solutions in these vignettes are simple to devise in clinical practice. A plan may appear obvious once it has been shown likely to work.

It is impossible to capture in a vignette the amount of time and work required for therapists to devise a neuropsychosocial treatment plan. There are often many false starts, because initial conceptualizations of the phenomenology of dyscontrol may miss an essential element. Moreover, neuropsychosocial treatment plans may change dramatically as they evolve. In vignettes they seem simple. However, the final neuropsychosocial environment that these vignettes present can take months in the real world to generate, test, refine, abandon, redevelop, implement, and finally settle upon. Furthermore, these vignettes highlight the development of certain elements in neuropsychosocial plans. In actual cases, neuropsychosocial plans can be more complex. The final vignette was constructed to portray the type of complexity therapists may encounter in more complete neuropsychosocial plans.

The following vignettes represent a composite picture of clinical scenarios. They draw upon an accumulation of clinical experience but do not reflect upon or represent any particular case or person with brain injury. It is important to realize that should these vignettes seem clinically similar to any real case therapists might see, therapists should not rely on the plans presented here, but rather on real plans from the real world. They should not be misled to think the vignettes are actual cases just because of similarities between these vignettes and their own cases. Similarities that appear are indicative of the commonality of human behavior after brain injury.

Vignette one

Scenario

A woman with brain injury presents with a history of severe physical aggression. Her aggression consists of punching people. She is quite strong and has hurt a number of people. She generally does not throw things or hit objects. She avoids raising her voice, as she is typically soft spoken. Her aggression appears to be unprovoked in that she might hit someone in the middle of an otherwise pleasant conversation. The other aspect of her behavioral dyscontrol is to wander into other people's rooms. She tends to get lost. The frequency of her aggression is high — she hits people more than five times an hour.

Procedure

In light of the immediacy of her dangerousness, therapists initiate strategies to ensure the safety of others. To address her wandering, they assign her a temporary one-to-one staffing level. The therapist assigned to her temporarily is responsible for redirecting her when she wanders towards someone else's room. Apart from the unpleasantness she may experience when she is lost, her therapists want to avoid having her enter someone else's room and then hit a person in that room.

Therapists institute a preliminary neuropsychosocial approach with regard to her physical aggression. They establish a "two step" rule for anyone who talks with her or stands close to her. That is, everyone must stand a distance of at least two strides from her so that if she initiates a punch there is time to step aside or to block the blow. In addition, whenever possible they place a chair or table between her and themselves. Furthermore, they invite her to sit down when they want to talk with her. Therapists determine never to be near her when they are seated and she is standing, because such a position makes them vulnerable.

This initial neuropsychosocial procedure provides therapists with increased safety to study the phenomenology of her aggression. Based upon their analysis they can develop a more comprehensive plan.

Phenomenology of dyscontrol

Over time, therapists observe a number of variables essential to understanding her aggression. First, she only hits during conversations in which she makes a request of a therapist and the request cannot be met. Typically a therapist told her "no" or used a variant thereof. She then rapidly strikes without warning. She is otherwise in control during conversations. Therapists observe that she avoids aggression at other times: she does not hit people as she walks by them or during activities if she has no unmet requests. In fact, she is very tolerant of redirection when therapists initiate it, such as when they redirect her to her room if they find her wandering.

Cognitive assessment reveals a very clear pattern of deficits. Her reasoning skills are adequate. However, she is highly distractible, she has severe memory deficits, and she is very impulsive.

Her therapists are able to come to some conclusions regarding her behavior. This woman exhibits aggression in a very specific manner. She is aggressive during conversations with therapists when she makes a request and the therapists say "no." She poses no risk to other persons with brain injury because she realizes (good reasoning skill) that they have no power to grant her requests. Indeed, she never even approaches other persons with brain injury to make requests. When told "no" by therapists, her response is immediate (impulsivity and disinhibition): she punches them. Her high rate of aggression is due to her frequent requests. Because she is unable to remember (severe memory deficit), she forgets that she asked and was denied her request only a few minutes before. In fact, she forgets that she hit someone earlier. Therefore she returns to make her request again and the cycle repeats itself.

She wanders into others' rooms because of her memory deficit. She accepts redirection easily because her aggression follows denial of her requests but does not result from offers of advice or guidance. While wandering may be a problem, in her case aggression is not a sequela to wandering since she tolerates therapists or others telling her to leave the room.

Neuropsychosocial plan

Therapists construct a behavioral plan for this woman based upon their observations of her phenomenology of dyscontrol and her cognitive functioning. First, the temporary one-to-one staff level is discontinued. Because this woman is pleasant and appropriate with other persons with brain injury and is never aggressive with them, she does not need the constant supervision to protect them from her.

Second, therapists place a large sign on her door with her name and photograph to help her orient to her room. The photograph of her is particularly helpful. Therapists later put items that she has made herself (e.g., collages) on her door to add further personal meaning. These personal items aid her with memory, because they are things that she has spent time making. Marking her door in this manner substantially decreases her wandering.

Third, because she only hits after asking for something she cannot have, therapists realize that they can use her memory deficit and distractibility to avoid aggression in these instances. They determine that when she makes a request, instead of saying the actual word "no," or a variant thereof, they can offer an alternative. When they do this, she forgets her initial request and proceeds with the alternative. For example, when she makes a request for candy that her health and diet prohibits, therapists might state, "Hey, let me see. I'd like to help with that. I can see what I can do. Would you like a glass of juice?" The first few sentences buy time for her to forget her request. Therapists then distract her with an alternative that she accepts. They never say the word "no" or "I'm sorry you can't have that" or other similar phrases.

This woman's memory deficit leads her to make repeated requests, but her memory problem accompanied by her distractibility lead to a neuropsychosocial treatment plan element. She will live in a world where people avoid saying "no" to her. This plan can generalize to a group home setting with therapists trained in its application. Of course, therapists must take care to fill all of her requests that they can meet. Therapists are aware that they should only follow this procedure when the requests are of such a nature that they cannot fulfill them.

Finally, this woman's aggression is not "unprovoked" as first thought. It occurs after a specific conversational pattern. Therapists can avoid the need to be constantly on guard with her since they can predict what will trigger aggression. However, since it remains uncertain when in conversation she will make a request, the two-step rule remains in her plan as a precaution in case a therapist slips and says "no" or a variant thereof. Also, to add an extra component of safety, therapists still stand to talk with her. However, therapists determine that keeping a table or chair between her and them is now excessive and unnecessary.

Result

This woman's level of aggression drops dramatically. She stops hitting. Her emotional state remains appropriate. She wanders less and can typically find her own room. She still accepts redirection as needed. She is able to live in a group home.

Vignette two

Scenario

Another woman with brain injury has a history of dangerous physical aggression. She assaults people, including family members. In addition, she attempts to manipulate other people and when this fails, she uses verbal intimidation. She demonstrates little regard for the effect her behavior has upon other people. Therapists who discuss this with her detect a cavalier attitude about the value she has for other people. She believes that intimidation, threats, and violence are acceptable tools to achieve what she wants.

Procedure

Therapists initially approach her with the intent of understanding her value system. They explore her perspectives and test these by studying her response to alternative viewpoints. She responds with surprise to the idea that she might achieve her goals through building relationships with other people or through compromise. She views these processes as inefficient and less effective in getting what she wants, and she rejects them.

Phenomonology of dyscontrol

Cognitive assessment reveals that this woman has reasonable abilities. She is able to attend. She can remember overall themes in information and can recall particular items in detail. Her verbal reasoning skills are good, but she may miss the larger picture and struggle with context. She can plan, up to a point. Finally, at times she shows some disinhibition and impulsivity.

Usually, self-interest motivates her. Her self-interest, however, focuses on short-term gain, often at long-term expense, but she fails to consider that in her decision making. In part, the tendency to favor short-term gain reflects her cognitive difficulties in that she can reason, but she misses context and the larger picture. Also, she acts in a short-sighted manner because of her disinhibition. It takes more time to think about the long term. Short-term gains and immediate gratification are her overriding approach.

This woman respects only those who are equally adept at getting their own way. Any presentation of weakness, which by her definition includes poor deal making or overt concern for others, is evidence that she should press harder to get what she wants to the point of making threats or using violence. Her value system is unalterable.

Neuropsychosocial plan

Therapists realize that all discussions with this woman are negotiations. Moreover, she will use anything therapists say as fodder for future negotiations. Thus, they note that a therapist can never say to another therapist in her presence "I'm not sure; let's go talk about it privately" because the woman would note that one of the therapists appeared unsure. In future interactions she might accuse that therapist of not being able to make decisions, and therefore she might refuse to deal with him or her. Rather, the therapist would say, "Let's go talk about it privately," or "I have an idea I want to compare with your ideas; let's go talk about it privately," whether or not the therapist is unsure or even has an idea. As a result, any interaction with this woman must entail her viewing the therapists in a position of strength, power, and assertiveness. However, if every therapist appears decisive, she will attempt to split them by presenting subtly different issues to each one so as to obtain conflicting agreements with different therapists. She will then attempt to assert the validity of the arrangement that she believes is most favorable to her. To prevent her from doing this, the therapists assign a lead therapist to negotiate all arrangements with his woman. All other therapists remain adamant about agreeing with the elements of the plan as negotiated by the lead therapist. They implement the plan according to the agreements made by the lead therapist. Of course, behind the scenes all of the therapists confer to help the lead therapist negotiate. With the woman with brain injury, the plan is not open to explanation or debate by other therapists and they do not allow her to engage them in discussions of the plan. In short, all other therapists are assertive and strong in their interactions with her in support of the plan. Therapists take all of her complaints to the lead therapist who consults all of the therapists behind the scenes on how to proceed with negotiations. There is team coordination.

Result

As a result this woman's episodes of behavioral dyscontrol drop dramatically. The lead therapist is a negotiator who has more skill than the woman possesses in negotiating. The woman respects this therapist. There is consistency across therapists, and within the scope of the role the plan assigns to them she views them as powerful and as having determination. She is behaviorally compliant because she has negotiated her privileges. In fact, her privileges are ones that the therapists can accept because of the skill of the lead therapist. Hence, her neuropsychosocial plan is to have a designated, exceptionally skillful negotiator for her to address and other assertive therapists who administer precisely the negotiated agreements. She is content because she negotiates her status, and the therapists are content because the negotiated status is reasonable from their perspective.

Vignette three

Scenario

A man with brain injury exhibits repeated aggression during episodes of behavioral dyscontrol. He physically assaults therapists or other persons with brain injury. He is capable of destroying property. His aggression can include verbal threats. He sometimes tries to intimidate other people.

Procedure

Therapists began the process of study necessary to construct a neuropsychosocial environment. He presents as disinhibited and resistant to redirection. He may acknowledge his behavioral dyscontrol up to a point and then becomes defensive and loses control again. He is labile and exhibits emotions ranging from inappropriate laughter to irritability. He challenges therapists physically and is particularly threatening because he is quick and powerful. He likes to stand very close to other people. In fact, when he is in a good mood, he will try to rest his arm across therapists' shoulders as if they were his buddies. He is highly confabulatory. He often relates long, convoluted stories in which he supposedly was in the military, in the mafia, or knew famous people. Typically, these stories establish him as a powerful person to be reckoned with, strengthening his sense of self-esteem. Efforts to have him reconsider these stories are met with aggression.

He can become demanding. When his demands are not met quickly, he becomes angry. He often begins with repeated demands and intrusiveness and then advances to threats and aggression. He exhibits these behaviors more frequently with those therapists he determines lack confidence or are afraid of him.

His interactions with other persons with brain injury often result in aggression. He attempts to socialize with them, but things always seem to go astray. He seems intolerant, but further study reveals that this initial impression of him by therapists is inaccurate. Rather, he is unable to handle the process of interacting with other people.

Despite his overall presentation, this man demonstrates notable positive attributes. He is motivated to do well. He is ashamed, at times, by his own behavior. He seems embarrassed by therapists' efforts to redirect him. He has an excellent sense of humor. He enjoys playing chess. He has a very supportive, concerned, and involved family, although he can say things that hurt them sometimes.

Cognitive assessment documents a number of deficits. These include impairments in visual processing (visual memory, visual perceptual reasoning, etc.), problem solving and flexibility, and impulse control. While his verbal skills are a relative strength, his verbal memory is impaired. His deficits correlate with therapists' clinical observations that he can converse, but that he is distractible and requires structure. Behaviorally, he is disinhibited and struggles to conceptualize alternative ways to proceed.

Therapists make an initial attempt to use insight-oriented psychotherapy, skill building, and the application of consequences. These techniques prove unsuccessful by themselves but reveal crucial aspects of his functioning for eventual inclusion in his neuropsychosocial treatment plan. He responds to traditional psychotherapy with very strong resistance. His need to maintain his self-image is sufficiently powerful that it restricts his willingness to examine his own behavior. This remains so despite much effort on the part of therapists to create a safe emotional world for him in which he can reflect on his behavior, providing reassurance, support, respect, and hope. Furthermore, when at times he shows periods of being able to self-reflect, his inability to tolerate his own emotional arousal during the process of self examination leads to escalation of dyscontrol.

This man's cognitive deficits interfere with skill building. Since he presents himself as having adequate skills, he shows little motivation for skill acquisition. Also, skill building requires tolerance of errors during skill acquisition, and he handles the emotions that accompany early learning trials poorly.

Implementing consequences following inappropriate behavior makes his behavior worse. When therapists withhold privileges, his behavior escalates. For example, when he is not allowed to go on an outing after aggression, his aggression increases.

Therapists become aware during their trials of these traditional techniques that this man is incapable of maintaining behavioral control if he experiences emotional arousal. Interestingly the emotions that lead to behavioral dyscontrol can be positive as well as negative. When he receives too much praise he can also lose behavioral control, because he may become expansive. In fact, when good things happen in his life that make him happy, the emotional arousal that they entail can lead to episodes of behavioral dyscontrol. Furthermore, he actively seeks arousal. If bored, he will trigger events so as to become aroused. His intent is not to lose control, but rather to stimulate himself.

Phenomenology of dyscontrol

This man's aggression is a result of cognitive impairment coupled with issues of self-esteem. He has difficulty processing nonverbal communication, and therefore can be socially inappropriate. His verbal communication is confounded by variable attention and distractibility. For example, he notes the emotional tone that accompanies verbal redirection, but misses the reasons why he receives therapists' directives. Moreover, he forgets what he has done after he acts inappropriately, and his impulsivity leads him to repeated interactions in which he can be intrusive, demanding, and inappropriate.

His low self-esteem also plays a role in his behavior. During his recollection of episodes of dyscontrol, he often positions himself as the victim of other peoples' inappropriate behavior. He explains his own dyscontrol as a reaction to their behavior, whereas in actuality he often instigates the events. His pride, however, requires him to maintain this erroneous viewpoint to facilitate his sense of self-worth. His value system, which does incorporate socially acceptable standards, is in sharp contrast to his behavior. His inaccurate recollection of events, however, permits him to continue his sense of self-esteem.

Emotional arousal triggers his behavior. Such arousal includes both seemingly positive and negative emotions. Despite his difficulty in handling arousal, he seeks it out. However, often too much exposure to emotion-inducing interactions leads to him losing control.

Neuropsychosocial plan

The plan for this man with brain injury addresses his cognitive, behavioral, and emotional functioning. It represents the culmination of therapists' knowledge about him that they acquired through observation, cognitive evaluation, and trials of treatment approaches. To start, therapists avoid the use of contingencies with him. As a result, therapists do not reward or withhold privileges based upon his behavior unless an immediate privilege is due and he is still out of control. For example, if he is set to go to the cafeteria and he is yelling or hitting, therapists may temporarily withhold the privilege of going to the cafeteria to ensure the safety of others. Once he is calm, however, he can then continue with his routine and make the trip. The trip to the cafeteria is not withheld because he was out of control earlier.

The lack of contingencies also applies when he hits another person. In the case of many persons with brain injury, therapists require that they have a time out in their room after they hit someone. Such a procedure in this man's case inflames him. Instead, when he hits someone, therapists suggest to him that he might consider going to his room to "get away from the hubbub," but indicate that it is his choice to do so. Therapists deliver this suggestion in a calm, neutral manner. With this approach, he typically voluntarily goes to his room. This approach allows him to calm himself, and he stops hitting. Otherwise, with contingences he becomes more aroused, rebels, and persists in his aggression.

It is crucial that when he is out of control, therapists give redirection without any emotional overtones. With other persons with brain injury, therapists might use a disapproving affect to accompany redirection after persons with brain injury are aggressive, to signal disapproval. In his case, therapists omit this feedback element since it triggers behavioral escalation. He accepts redirection better when therapists are emotionally neutral.

In the same way they avoid negative consequences for behavioral dyscontrol, therapists take care to measure the amount of positive regard he receives so that they avoid excessively arousing him. Once he is aroused, even by positive emotions, a negative thought or event that he might otherwise tolerate leads to behavioral dyscontrol, because he must process it while he is emotionally charged. In his case, it does not matter that the original arousal is a result of positive events, praise, or attention.

The plan for him emphasizes a flat affect whenever therapists give him instruction or redirection. When given the time to calm, he will do so if there are no further arousing stimuli. The more agitated he becomes, the more important that it is for therapists to be "dead calm."

Therapists must carefully monitor their body language, facial expressions, and tone of voice around him when he becomes agitated. Otherwise, he will feed on their frustration or disapproval, which will incite him. When therapists avoid showing irritation, he calms. In fact, at times when he threatens physical aggression against therapists, the best approach for them is to stand calmly, blending into the wall, saying nothing, letting him gather himself together, permitting him to calm.

Therapists withhold him from participating in group treatment or interactions because he is unable to maintain behavioral control during groups. He cannot handle the dynamics of group processes. If the group discusses his problems and limitations, whether it requires him to self-disclose or hear the observations of other persons with brain injury, he escalates emotionally and loses control. If the group members focus on positive aspects of his functioning, he absorbs the energy of so much attention and then loses control. If the conversation is too subtle or ignores him, he becomes bored and seeks stimulation. He may make inflammatory comments or begin to tell other people what they should do. When they respond, he loses control.

Therapists do provide controlled levels of individual stimulation for this man. Otherwise, he becomes intrusive as he seeks stimulation. He can easily annoy other persons with brain injury and he may inflame their emotions. To avoid his provoking other persons with brain injury, therapists provide him with opportunities for conversation or other activities.

A particularly useful activity for this man is playing chess. He knew how to play chess before onset and takes pride in knowing how to play. He appreciates that chess is a difficult game. As such, he tolerates losing games as part of the culture of chess. Of particular relevance is the fact that he remains calm when playing chess even as he loses pieces or games. Therapists find that while he is playing chess he can even tolerate conversation on difficult topics, such as his behavior. Therefore, when therapists do need to give him feedback or raise topics that might irritate him, doing so during a game of chess is often the most productive time to proceed with the dialogue.

It is interesting to note here the uses of chess not only as part of the plan for this man, but also as a tool in the care of other persons with brain injury. In many cases of brain injury, therapists who are expert chess players can clinically detect cognitive dysfunction among persons with brain injury through the use of chess. By playing chess with them, therapists can see errors in their attention, planning, sequencing, memory, and visuospatial processing. If therapists are good enough to manipulate the chess game, then they can play the game to create opportunities to observe particular deficits. Lebow notes the diagnostic and therapeutic use of chess with other populations also.[1]

In addition to remaining calm while playing chess, this man demonstrates calmness when visiting with members of the clergy. He tends to be respectful of them when they visit. He is able to converse with them without behavioral escalation, and is cooperative and deferential. He conceptualizes them as different from the members of his treatment team and will accept their reflections on his behavior. Moreover, he accepts their role in setting standards. Thus, his plan includes visits from the clergy to help him explore behavioral expectations.

When therapists must redirect him, they make a special effort to conduct such discussions in private. If he escalates in a public space where other people are present, whether they are therapists or other persons with brain injury, therapists invite him to accompany them to a private place to "help them meet *their* needs," rather than telling him to come with them because of his behavior. Telling him in front of someone he has hit that he has to go with the therapists to review this episode leads to escalation. For this reason, therapists do not say to him, "Fred, we have to go to your room to discuss your hitting Tom." Instead, they might say "Hey, Fred, I need to talk with you about something. Can you join me away from this chaos? Let's go talk somewhere. How about your room?"

The principle in effect is to avoid lowering of this man's self-esteem. He perceives redirection as shameful. When it is done anywhere that others might overhear, he becomes defensive. This defensiveness leads to assertion of his behavioral correctness, blaming of others, resistance, arousal, and further aggression. Of course, it is inappropriate for therapists to reflect publicly on behavior of any person with brain injury, though public redirection to desist behavior is sometimes necessary. In the case of this man, however, the preceding procedure proves most effective. If therapists reflect on his behavior in private, without time pressure, he can at times accept his own role in events. His therapists recognize that this private discourse is a slow process and is usually only successful with therapists he knows well and trusts. Private conversation, without pressure for him to take responsibility, engaged in slowly by therapists with whom he has rapport, makes him more receptive to suggestions. This process decreases his arousal.

Regardless of when therapists engage him regarding his behavior, it is important that they utilize a non-confrontational style. Statements that begin with "you," such as "You shouldn't ...," agitate him. In contrast, statements that start with "I," such as "I am disappointed that ..." are less accusatory, and he tolerates the discussion better than he does when therapists are more direct. The guiding principle is to examine his behavior in terms of its impact on how therapists or others feel following his behavior. The goal is not to increase his guilt, however. Instead, the intent is to support him in his efforts to control his behavior better and thereby have better relationships with other people. Therapists attend to the fact that he does show concern for other people. The message that he can influence how others feel is empowering for him.

Therapists do best when providing guidance for this man if they first gain his respect. To do so, they must demonstrate to him a combination of confidence in their own abilities and perspectives accompanied by respect for his input. He will reject therapists who have a style that is too dictatorial, as well as therapists who are insecure or hesitant. If he senses that therapists are afraid of him, he will challenge them. In addition, he responds poorly to therapists who are overly formal, although therapists must avoid attempting to become his friend, ignoring boundary issues.

Therapists must maintain a balanced approach with him. This is most necessary when he strives to enhance his self-esteem by being "macho." Therapists will find it therapeutic to permit him to position himself as a dominant individual up to a point, as long as he does not progress to behavioral manifestations of that attitude. If his verbal assertions that he is a "force to be reckoned with" become too assertive, therapists can deflect him by changing topics.

For the most part, this man's verbal claims make him feel important and are harmless. His declarations about his history often take on a confabulatory flavor. These stories build his sense of self-worth. They often involve long, convoluted tales about who he knows and what he has done. His role ranges from being powerful and heroic to being secretive sometimes and infamous at other times. Therapists can distract him and redirect him when he relates a confabulatory story without challenging its veracity. In fact, contradicting his recollections will lead to his becoming increasingly more intense about his remembrances, heading him toward aggression.

When therapists relate well to him he can attempt to become too familiar. He may stand too close and unintentionally violate therapists' personal space. He does accept the concept of needing to stand 3 feet away, or at arm's length, during conversations, but he forgets it. However, he tolerates reminders about this requirement and will readily step back when therapists ask him to do so. Therapists can aid him by slowly extending their arm toward him in a horizontal position to measure the appropriate interpersonal distance that he needs to maintain. However, it is critical that therapists do this with palm down and flat, not vertical and facing toward him. Palm down represents measuring distance and is friendly to him; palm up and facing him (the "stop" position) is offensive to him. Precision counts. Therapists who fail to gently assert their personal space in this manner may find that they have backed all the way across a room when interacting with him, as they step back to increase interpersonal space and he steps forward to close it up.

When this man forgets to keep an arm's length away, he sometimes also places his arm over therapists' shoulders and neck. In addition to this being a violation of personal space, it places therapists in a vulnerable position; it is also physically uncomfortable. However, if therapists move their arm closest to him and slip it under his arm and across his neck and shoulders, his arm will harmlessly slide off their shoulders and down their back. This movement allows them to step away, turn toward him, and reestablish arm's length distance between the two of them. Therapists can do this without calling attention to their maneuver and without any verbal comment on their part. Their behavior controls the interaction without any risk of escalation on his part. If therapists must explicitly discuss his tendency to put his arm on their shoulders and neck, they can emphasize his size and strength as to why they are uncomfortable in this position. He responds well to this explanation.

At times, this man displays an excellent sense of humor. He will joke and tease appropriately. Therapists can respond in a like manner. In fact, therapists can disarm him when he is irritable or resistant to redirection by using humor. As with all aspects of interaction with him, therapists must take care that their use of humor and the style of their humor match his level of functioning, is therapeutic, is not derogatory, and is acceptable to him. When therapists use humor effectively with him, it can dissipate his frustration.

In contrast to how therapists respond to him when he is confabulatory, they can be more directive when he loses track of what he wishes to say. Sometimes he hesitates in the middle of a sentence and then proceeds in an unrelated, tangential direction. In such instances, he needs assistance in returning to his original train of thought. Otherwise, he may become frustrated because he never communicated a point that was important to him. Later on, he can become angry with therapists who fail to meet his expectations when in reality he never completely explained his concerns. When therapists return him to his point in conversation they decrease the likelihood of future aggression.

A particular frustration for him is when therapists ask him to wait before they address his requests. He has considerable difficulty with delay of gratification. Experience shows that he may be able to wait a couple of minutes, but rarely more than 5 minutes, and almost never 10 minutes. When therapists ask him to monitor a clock so he can judge how long he is waiting, he may do so, but this procedure does little to decrease his impatience. After a few minutes he will repeat his request, becoming increasingly more intrusive and agitated. For this reason it is best for therapists to be available to review his requests as they occur and, most importantly, to anticipate them. Therapists' insight into the pattern of his desires allows them to be proactive. Furthermore, therapists find that it is beneficial to assign one therapist to take the lead in managing his requests so that consistency increases. His difficulty with delay of gratification worsens when different therapists require him to wait different periods of time.

This man's difficulty in waiting also has an impact on how therapists manage episodes of behavioral dyscontrol. When therapists suggest that he go to his room after behavioral episodes, they need to specify a short amount of time for him to be in his room. Otherwise, as his impatience grows he will exit his room prematurely, triggering their demanding that he comply with their time period. This then escalates his behavior.

The last element in this man's behavior plan involves his relationship with his family. His family is very important to him, and family members have been very supportive. He enjoys visits with them. They go on outings with him into the community, and he looks forward to these trips. Because of his enjoyment of these visits, therapists and family members work to schedule them. Therapists and his family take care to limit the duration of these visits, however; when he becomes too excited, even while experiencing positive emotions, he can lose behavioral control. In the case of family visits, the behavioral dyscontrol may occur after the visit rather than during the visit. His family is a sufficiently powerful influence that he usually maintains control while he is with them.

Result

The construction of the plan for this person requires extensive observation and contemplation by innovative therapists. His plan is complex, but experienced therapists are able to conceptualize and implement it. As the therapists devise and add plan elements over time, his behavior improves. Community reentry becomes a reality.

Conclusions

The transition for therapists from theoretical understanding of neuropsychosocial case conceptualization to translation of theory into concrete behavioral plans, and then to clinical skill in implementing plans, can be challenging. The neuropsychosocial approach will likely be most useful to therapists for their previously least successful and most dangerous cases. Therapists can become as adept with the neuropsychosocial approach as they are with other treatment processes, but they must keep in mind that because they are applying it to their most difficult cases, the hurdles they must overcome for success are higher. Therapists commonly have more training and experience with insight-oriented, skill-building, and contingency management therapies. As they acquire expertise with neuropsychosocial treatment, their comfort level will increase and their outcomes will improve. They will find that this approach greatly complements other courses of treatment on easier cases, as well.

In summary, the creation of a neuropsychosocial environment, supplemented by innovative medication management, permits therapists to successfully treat even severe behavioral dysfunction after acquired brain injury. Persons with brain injury who otherwise would be restrained, medicated into a stupor, jailed, or committed to state hospitals, can live in the community. The opportunity that the neuropsychosocial treatment approach affords therapists to save the lives of persons with brain injury is amazingly rewarding for therapists and life changing for persons with brain injury.

Reference

1. Lebow, A., Personal communication, 2002.

index

A

B

C

D

E

F

G

H

I

J

K

L

M

N

O

P

R

S

T

U

V

W